I0438755

Copyright
Alzheimer's Tips you Really Should Know

Alzheimer's Tips You Should Know

A must have guide for every caregiver family and friend of someone with Alzheimer's disease.

Angela V. Blackman

"They may forget your name, but they will never forget how you made them feel."

Maya Angelou

Table of Contents

Alzheimer's Tips You Should Know

Alzheimer's Tips You Should Know

INTRODUCTION

<u>**Alzheimer's disease**</u> affects millions of families all over the world and it is expected that over the next ten years more and more families will be touched by this disease. When it will strike and which family will be affected, no one knows.

In the face of a disease that damages the brain and affects almost every function of the body, many families and friends find the tasks of caregiving to be a major challenge.

As a caregiver to my mother who has had Alzheimer's disease for the last nine years, I understand the challenges, frustrations, emotional, social and physical stress that caregiving can have on an individual.

This book was written with the objective to make life easier for persons with Alzheimer's

Alzheimer's Tips You Should Know

disease, their families, friends and caregivers. In it you will find tips and strategies that will help you cope with the day to day challenges that you may face. Challenges such as bathing, nutrition, mealtime, what to do if you want to travel with your loved one, how to communicate at the time when speech becomes jumbled, how to keep your loved one active and engaged in the early middle and late stages of this disease and even how to deal with the messy issues that drive you crazy.

What is Alzheimer's disease

Alzheimer's is a disease of the brain, where cells degenerate and die causing a decline in memory and mental function. As the damage worsens, gradually there is a progressive loss of social and intellectual skills which can severely affect the day-to-day life of the person with the disease.

AREAS OF THE BRAIN AFFECTED BY ALZHEIMER'S DISEASE

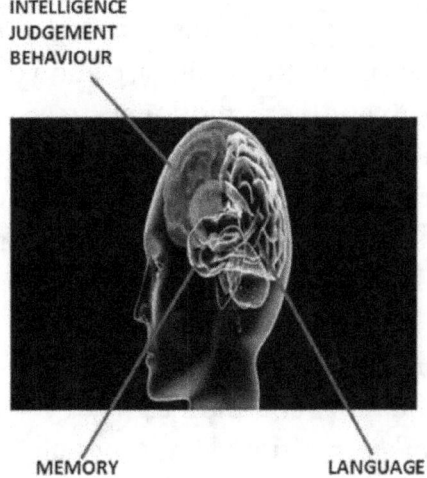

Alzheimer's Tips You Should Know

SIGNS and SYMPTOMS

If you notice these signs in your loved one, you should consult the doctor immediately. **Early diagnosis** of the disease can save you, your loved one with the disease and your family from conflict, emotional stress and pain in the long run. It also allows you and your loved one to plan for their future care, before they lose their ability to communicate clearly.

MEMORY LOSS

One of the most common signs of Alzheimer's is memory loss, especially forgetting recently learned information. Others include forgetting important dates or events; asking for the same information over and over; increasingly needing to rely on memory aids (e.g., reminder notes or electronic devices) or family members for things they used to handle on their own.

CHALLENGES PLANNING OR SOLVING PROBLEMS

Some people may experience changes in their ability to develop and follow a plan or work with numbers. They may have trouble following a familiar recipe or keeping track of monthly bills. They may have difficulty concentrating and take much longer to do things than they did before.

DIFFICULTY COMPLETING FAMILIAR TASKS

People with Alzheimer's often find it hard to complete daily tasks. Sometimes, people may have trouble driving to a familiar location, managing a budget at work or remembering the rules of a favorite game.

CONFUSION WITH TIME AND SPACE

People with Alzheimer's can lose track of dates, seasons and the passage of time. They may have trouble understanding something if it is not happening immediately. Sometimes they may forget where they are or how they got there.

Trouble understanding visual images and spatial relationships

For some people, having vision problems is a sign of Alzheimer's. They may have difficulty reading, judging distance and determining color or contrast, which may cause problems with driving.

New problems with words in speaking or writing

People with Alzheimer's may have trouble following or joining a conversation. They may stop in the middle of a conversation and have no idea how to continue or they may repeat themselves. They may struggle with vocabulary, have problems finding the right word or call things by the wrong name (e.g., calling a "watch" a "hand-clock")

Misplacing things and losing the ability to retrace steps

A person with Alzheimer's disease may put things in unusual places. They may lose things and be unable to go back over their steps to find them again. Sometimes, they may accuse others of stealing. This may occur more frequently over time.

Decreased or poor judgment

People with Alzheimer's may experience changes in judgment or decision-making. For example, they may use poor judgment when dealing with money, giving large amounts to telemarketers. They may pay less attention to grooming or keeping themselves clean.

Withdrawal from work or social activities

A person with Alzheimer's may start to remove themselves from hobbies, social activities, work projects or sports. They may have trouble keeping up with a favorite sports team or remembering how to complete a favorite hobby. They may also avoid being social because of the changes they have experienced.

Changes in mood and personality

The mood and personalities of people with Alzheimer's can change. They can become confused, suspicious, depressed, fearful or anxious. They may be easily upset at home, at work, with friends or in places where they are out of their comfort zone.

Referenced from: Alzheimer's Association

Stages of Alzheimer's Disease

Mild Alzheimer's disease

Alzheimer's disease is often first diagnosed in the mild or early stage, when it becomes clear to family and doctors, that the person is having significant trouble with memory and thinking.

In the mild Alzheimer's stage, people may

Forget where they put everyday things
The person may put things away and totally forget where they placed them. Sometimes they may even accuse you and others of theft or become suspicious.
Get lost
Your loved one may go shopping or for a routine walk but may become confused and find it difficult to return home.
Have trouble with complex tasks,

You may notice that your loved one is finding difficulty paying their bills or planning events.
Have trouble coming up with the right words sometimes
Your loved one may have problems saying the right words and carrying on conversations.
Feel less social or moody
You may find that the person withdraws him/herself from social events that they once enjoyed. This may be because they realize that something is changing in their life and may have feelings of embarrassment.

Mild Alzheimer's can last for years. The person may be able to live independently throughout this stage but they will need a lot of support from family and friends.

To make daily life easier, try these tips:

Provide a notebook and encourage them to write down important information such as names, phone numbers, appointments, and their address to carry around with them.

Encourage them to make "to do" lists and reminder notes, and label cupboards with words or pictures to remind them of what is inside.

Call to remind them of things like meal and medication times or purchase a <u>pill</u> <u>dispenser with automatic reminders.</u>

Encourage the person to join a support group where they can talk about how Alzheimer's affects their life and learn how other people are dealing with it.

At this stage the person should exercise, limit alcohol, and stay involved in activities they enjoy.

Moderate Alzheimer's disease

During the moderate or middle stage of Alzheimer's disease, the person may become more confused and forgetful and begin to need help with daily activities and self-care.

This is the longest stage of Alzheimer's. It can last many years -- it's different from person to person. As Alzheimer's progresses the person's memory will get worse and they will have more difficulty with language and thinking clearly.

At this stage they may:

Not always know family and friends

At this stage the person may begin to forget family and friends. They may be able to call names but be unable to connect the name with the person.

Lose track of times and places

Your loved one may lose track of the time of the day, and the days of the week and also where they are at one point or the other.

Forget details in their life

The person may forget their address, phone number, or where they went to high school or college or other personal information.

Have problems dressing and undressing (click here for tips on dealing with this)

The person may have trouble putting clothes on in the right order or picking the right clothes, and later bathing and using the toilet

Jumble words

As the disease progresses your loved one will gradually lose their ability to communicate and may jumble their words.

Have poor judgment

At this stage your loved one will lose the ability to make sound decisions about their health, finances, or safety.

In some instances the person may also:

See or hear things that aren't there

Suspect people of lying, cheating, or stealing from you

Be depressed or anxious

Become angry or violent

When Alzheimer's is at the moderate stage your loved one will probably need to live with family or in a residential care setting, or have a trained caregiver in their home. They may need help to get dressed, take medicines safely, and manage their finances. It may be unsafe for them to use the kitchen and be alone.

Severe Alzheimer's disease

In the severe or late stage of Alzheimer's, the person's mental and physical functions continue to decline.

They may experience the following:

Inability to speak
Communication skills will be severely affected as the person finds it difficult to speak and also understand what you are saying.

Decreased mobility
Your loved one may need help walking and later be unable to sit up, smile, or hold up their head.

Incontinence
They may have trouble controlling their bowels or bladder.

Wandering
At this stage wandering is very possible and the person may get lost.

Habits

Your loved one may have habits like wringing hands, shredding tissues, seeing things that are not there and pulling things apart.

When Alzheimer's is in the severe stage, the brain is unable to tell the body what to do. Therefore the person may sit on the toilet, forgetting what to do there, or hold food in their mouth, not remembering how to swallow.

In the late stages the person will need 24 hour care as they will need help with most daily activities and personal care.

Caring for someone with Alzheimer's disease is a journey that will require compassion, love and an enormous amount of patience. It also requires knowledge and information, if you are to effectively care for your loved one and yourself. As you read the following chapters of this book, you will find tips and strategies, which are intended to make life easier for caregiver and care receiver. Remember, however, strategies are not fail-proof and what may work for one person may not have the same effect on another. Never stop trying.

"You can complain because roses have thorns or you can rejoice because thorns have roses" ZIGGY

Activities for Early,middle and late stages of Alzheimer's disease

You will find that as Alzheimer's disease progresses, your loved one will gradually lose the ability to do several things that once came easy. This may become a painful and emotional process for you and your loved one, as you see their demise from stage to stage. However, the loss of regular function does not mean that there is nothing that can be done. There are several activities that can engage and stimulate you and your loved one as you take this journey together.

How to choose an activity

When looking for activities, try to use those that are stage appropriate. That is, activities that can be used dependent on whether the person is in the early, middle or late stage and what their abilities are.

Consider the interests and hobbies of the individual. Think about the things that they liked to do before Alzheimer's. Maybe it was gardening, building things, flower arranging, taking walks, watching movies or even dancing. Though you will have to make adjustments accordingly, you can use these as ways to keep your loved one active.

Choose activities that can be shared by family and friends. There is not every activity that you can share because of time constraints, but wherever possible try to make time for the family to share in activities with the person who has Alzheimer's disease. This brings a sense of normalcy to the family and also serves as a stress reducer for everyone.

Alzheimer's Tips You Should Know

Choose simple activities that provide a connection with everyday activities of life, such as folding clothes, arranging flowers, gardening or even dusting furniture.

Observe the response to the activities: whether the person enjoys them or if they are creating frustration. If they are frustrating for the individual do not continue, try something else.

Encourage and praise your loved one for their successes and do not blame them for failures that may occur.

EARLY STAGE ACTIVITIES

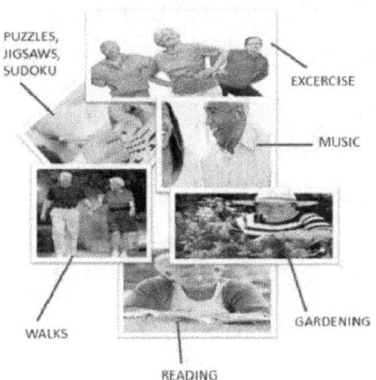

PUZZLES, JIGSAWS, SUDOKU

EXCERCISE

MUSIC

WALKS

GARDENING

READING

Activities for the early stages

In the early stages of Alzheimer's disease, your loved one may still be able to engage in activities as normal. At this stage, keeping their brains stimulated is a good idea. **Puzzles, trivia, word search** and such like, are good activities to use, however, if you find your loved one becoming agitated, or stressed, you should discontinue.

Alzheimer's Tips You Should Know

When choosing activities for or participating with your loved one bear in mind the following changes that may have occurred during this stage.

The person may have:

Impaired logic and sequencing, when telling a story or joke.

They may use words incorrectly or make up some words.

May have what may appear to be inappropriate mood swings

Lack of motivation and be inattentive.

Difficulty carrying on a conversation and finishing sentences.

Gets lost, even in familiar places

Diminished physical abilities, balance, strength

Repeats questions or statements

May begin to misplace, lose, or hide things

It is a myth that people with Alzheimer's disease can do nothing. People with Alzheimer's disease need to be active and do things they enjoy. As caregivers, family and friends we must focus on their current abilities and don't expect too much. Simple things like planning and knowing what to do each day may be troublesome for them and they may become fearful and worried, or quiet and withdrawn. If this happens remember that the person may just need a hand getting started.

In the early stages your loved one may still be able to function as normal and may be able to engage in regular activities.

Have conversations about what's happening at home and around the world. Talk about the good things that are happening in the family and stories of the past that they enjoyed.

Alzheimer's Tips You Should Know

During this stage the person may start to feel a sense of confusion about certain things and they may find it difficult to read printed books on their own. However, they can still enjoy a good novel by listening to **audio books.**

Play music and watch movies together. However, if you find that the person is becoming irritable or agitated you should change to something else.

Household chores

Allow the person to continue doing as much as they can for themselves, but monitor them carefully so that you can pick up any changes in their abilities. For example, you may notice that dishes are piling up in the sink or they may start wearing the same shirt without it being laundered. This does not mean that they are being lazy or dirty but that they are forgetting how to perform these tasks. You may not need to take over but offer some assistance.

Cooking and Baking

In the early stages your loved one may still be able to cook and bake. However, this activity should be carefully monitored to make sure that they can continue cooking safely. Cooking can be very dangerous for persons with Alzheimer's disease as the person may forget to turn off the stove, they may cook in plastic containers or they may even place newspapers or other flammable material on the fire.

If the person can no longer cook or bake on their own they can still help you in the kitchen.

They may still enjoy:

Deciding what is needed to prepare the
dish
Making the dish
Measuring, mixing and pouring
Telling you how to prepare a dish
Tasting the food
Watching you or others cook
Don't forget to say "thank you"

Activities with Family and Children

Having family, friends and children around
can be an enjoyable experience for the person
with Alzheimer's disease. This can be a good
opportunity for them to talk and recall happy
memories and also create a loving
environment.

There are a number of things that you can do
together like: reading stories, playing board
games, walk in the park, go to sports or

Alzheimer's Tips You Should Know

school events that involve young people and talk about fond memories from childhood.

Sometimes just sitting and chatting with each other is one of the best activities you can do together.

Music and Dancing

When music is used in the correct way it can change moods, manage agitation and generate positive interaction.

Music brings back memories for all of us and throughout every stage of Alzheimer's disease playing music for your loved one is a good option. Music can soothe and relax and also create joy and excitement. Never mind the person may not remember the lyrics they will still enjoy their old favorites in jazz, gospel, r&b or whatever genre they liked. Some people feel the rhythm and may want to dance. Others enjoy listening to or talking about their favorite music. So, play their favorite CDs, tapes and records, sing and dance or enjoy a concert together. Go out dancing or dance in the house.

Please note that if the person says that they do not like the music or they become agitated or show by body language that they do not want to hear the music then you should turn it off.

Pets

Many people question whether giving a person with Alzheimer's disease a pet is a good idea. The people suited to answer that question are those who know the person best. You should ask yourself these questions:

Does the person love having animals around?

Are they allergic to any animals?

If your loved one never liked having animals around, then now is definitely not a good time to get one.

If the person suffers from allergies as result of animals being around, then the answer is also definitely no.

However, if the person enjoys pets then you have to determine which pet they would prefer. If communicating is difficult and asking them will not help, then use their past as a guide,

Did they prefer dogs or cats?
If the person preferred cats then having a cat may be a good idea. You need to ensure that whichever pet you choose that it is one that your loved one can handle, that it is loving and friendly and it is properly cleaned and fed.

For a person who enjoys animals having a pet may help them feel more loved and less

Alzheimer's Tips You Should Know

worried and also have a sense of belonging. Animals offer affection and love that is unconditional. It does not matter that the person has Alzheimer's disease, they will love them anyway. They also give the person an opportunity to get involved in meaningful activities such as feeding, grooming and walking or they can be good companions just sitting in the person's lap. They also provide sensory stimulation as the person strokes the fur as in the case of cats and dogs or visual stimulation as they watch fish in an aquarium.

Gardening

For a person who is still able gardening is an activity that has several benefits. It provides an opportunity for exercise and for the person to be outdoors. It also stimulates the senses and is another way to keep your loved one active and to maintain as normal a life as possible. The person can take care of the plants, plant flowers and vegetables and water the plants.

However, you must be watchful as persons with Alzheimer's disease are may wander away. You should also ensure the person wears gloves and boots.

Activities for middle stages

As your loved one enters the middle stage of Alzheimer's disease their declining abilities will become more evident. Though they may still be strong physically, you may notice a lack of interest or a decline in their ability to participate in mental and social activities. Games such as puzzles, trivia and reading may become more confusing and difficult for them to do. At this time you may need to engage in more physically oriented activities that they are capable of doing. However, you should still continue with the brain activities that they can handle, for as long as possible.

At some stage your loved one will reach the stage where they can only follow simple, clear directions and you will have to make adjustments accordingly. It is at this point, that you will find familiar **physical activities** less frustrating to the individual.

Physical Activities in the early and middle stages

As long as your loved one is still able you should get them involved in physical activities that are suitable to them. Think about what they enjoy doing and engage in it at a level that they can handle. Being active and getting exercise will help you and the person with Alzheimer's disease feel better.

Exercise helps keep the muscles, joints, and heart in good shape. It will also help them stay at a healthy weight. Exercising together would be more enjoyable and of course, it also keeps the person with Alzheimer's disease safe.

Even though you want the person to be independent for as much as possible, you also need to make sure that the person is safe when active. Remember there is always the possibility that the person may wander and never be found.

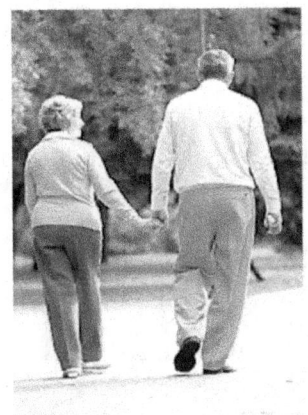

Alzheimer's Tips You Should Know

Getting started with physical exercise

Consult your doctor

Be realistic about how much activity can be done at one time.

Even though it's good to get an exercise routine going. Remember that it must be done at the pace that the person with Alzheimer's can handle. Let go of unrealistic expectations. They may not be able to walk like before or play a game of tennis according to the rules.Just enjoy.

Take a walk together as often as possible

Taking walks outdoors, as long as your loved one is able has several benefits for you and the person with Alzheimer's disease. Apart from the physical exercise it can also stimulate the senses.

Sense of Smell

To smell the fragrant flowers, the rain-soaked ground and other beautiful fragrances of the outdoors will stimulate your loved ones sense of smell and can have a calming effect.

Sense of Touch

There are so many textures outdoors to stimulate the sense of touch. Leaves, tree barks, twigs, petals, stones, sand and virtually anything can stimulate the sense of touch. Every solid object has texture, temperature, shape and could be rough or smooth, hard or soft and hot ,cold, warm or at room temperature Anything that we can touch or anything that touches us can be stimulating..**(Ensure that the objects are clean and safe))**

Sense of Sight

Outside there are many different and wonderful things to see: animals, birds, and green leafy plants, the sky, clouds, the sun and

Alzheimer's Tips You Should Know

other people. This is so much better than being isolated in the house. A change of scenery is good for your loved one and yourself. It can be helpful in reducing stress and calming aggressive behavior. However, you should avoid crowded and noisy environments as this can cause confusion and agitation in the person with Alzheimer's disease.

Sense of Hearing

Taking a walk outdoors can stimulate the sense of hearing. Our ability to hear provides us with a vibrant source of sensory stimulation. Auditory stimulation for people with Alzheimer's and dementia is effective for mood enhancement, relaxation, and cognition. The sound of the wind rustling through leaves or birds singing in the trees can be very effective. However, you should avoid loud, scary sounds as these may cause agitation

Outdoor activities can help alleviate symptoms of Alzheimer's, dementia, stress, and depression and improve cognitive function.

If you cannot go outdoors you can check your local TV guide to see if there are programs to help older adults exercise, or look for such videos online. Adding music to the exercises might help the person with Alzheimer's disease. Be selective and play music that they enjoy.

Dancing is another form of physical exercise that might keep your loved one happy, especially if it was something they enjoyed in the past. Play the music they loved and they may still enjoy a dance.

Break exercises into simple, easy-to-follow steps.

Remember, this is not an aerobics class where every routine is in sync; neither are you training for a marathon. Your loved one cannot handle tedious exercise. Do not expect them to get it all right,the whole aim is to keep them active. Also remember that at this

stage their ability to communicate and
understand instructions may be very impaired,
therefore you should be patient and give
simple instructions breaking the exercises
down step by step.

Comfortable shoes, clothing and liquids

Make sure the person's shoes and clothes are
comfortable and fit well and that they drink
water or juice after exercise.

As the disease progresses the person may not
be able to get around well. This presents more
challenges for the caregiver along with the
facts that the person may have trouble with
endurance, poor coordination, sore feet or
muscles, depression or illness other than
Alzheimer's disease. Some people may simply
have no interest at all in physical activities..

Even if the person has trouble walking or
face the challenges mentioned above they may
still be able to do:

Household chores

As with the early stages your loved one may still be able to do simple task around the house like sweeping and dusting, folding clothes and maybe a little gardening. They may not be able to complete the tasks on their own and might need more supervision than in the early stage. At this stage it may be a better idea to let them help you while you are doing these chores instead of leaving them to do it alone. It will give them something to do and maintain a measure of self-esteem.

Cooking and baking

During the moderate or middle stage of Alzheimer's disease, the person may become increasingly confused and forgetful and will need more help with daily activities and self-care. The person should not be allowed to continue cooking and baking on their own, but they could still help with deciding what is needed to prepare the dish, making the dish measuring, mixing and pouring, telling you how to prepare a dish, tasting the food or watching you or others cook if their current abilities allow. Remember that stages can last for years and affects people differently so that, what one person with Alzheimer's can do at a particular stage another person may not be able to do. **Don't forget to say "thank you"**

Activities with Family, Friends and Children

As the disease progresses, your loved one will experience drastic changes in personality and increased forgetfulness and confusion. When this occurs your loved one may become agitated and aggressive for seemingly no good reason. A normally mild and quiet person may shout at a child, friend or family member or become verbally abusive. This can be frightening especially for children. It is important that you be open and honest with the child explaining to them the effects of the disease and why granny or granddaddy is acting that way. It is also important for adults to get as much information as possible about the disease. The reality is that some family and friends may eventually drift away because of the aggression and accusations.

That aside having family, friends and children around is always good for the person with Alzheimer's disease and if their current abilities allow they may continue reading stories, playing board games, walk in the park, go to sports or school events that involve young people and talk about fond memories from childhood. When playing games at this stage the focus should not be on the rules just on having fun.

Music and Dancing

"Where words fail music speaks" Hans Christian Anderson

Listening to music is an activity that can be used throughout every stage of Alzheimer's disease. As with the early stage it can be used to reduce agitation and change moods not only for the care-receiver but also the caregiver.

In the middle stage you can play music or sing with the person, use music in the background to enhance the mood for both care giver and care receiver. It is better to use familiar relaxing music at this stage.

Please note that if the person says that they do not like the music or they become agitated or show by body language that they do not want to hear the music then you should turn it off.

If your loved one's current abilities permit the person can still dance to their favorite music.

Alzheimer's Tips You Should Know

Continue to play games, however, do not focus on the rules, just play and enjoy.
Playing games will keep them engaged, reduce boredom and help them to feel normal and independent.

Games you may try in the middle stages

<u>Jigsaw Puzzles with fewer and larger pieces</u>

<u>Qwirkle and other games</u>

> When having activities with persons in the middle stage remember that not every day will be the same do not force them to participate and do not overdo. It is important that you bear in mind your loved one's current abilities and remember that at this stage they may experience the following and these may influence their behaviors.

Sequencing and logic may become more and more impaired
They may not be able to find the right words and may make some up.

May become moody and have a change in personality so don't be upset if in the middle of an activity they became agitated.

They may neglect their hygiene and this could affect their social life.

The person's memory loss may become more obvious.

Inappropriate social behavior

Sleep disorders, including disruptions in the sleep/wake cycle and **sundowning***

The person may also lose the ability to read and write and therefore be unable to participate in certain activities. Their ability to understand rules of games may be lost and you should not expect them to play games according to the rules.

Activities for late stages

At this stage your loved ones abilities will be even more limited. However, this does not mean that they should be left to just sit in a chair. If your loved one can still use their hands, you can provide sensory balls, **activity pillows**, and other similar products that would keep them moving.

When doing these activities remember that at this stage your loved one may:

Have lost the ability to communicate verbally.

Alzheimer's Tips You Should Know

Need help with all activities of daily living.
Have lost more of their physical abilities and become less mobile
Become unresponsive to stimuli

Play calm relaxing music during the day, it's good for you and your care receiver. **Audio books** can also be used at this stage. If you are watching movies, avoid those with violence. Use **nature CD'S and DVD'S that are calming.**

Have a collection of old favorite music available to play.
Do sing-alongs, with tunes that they enjoyed singing in the past, like hymns, choruses or other songs they enjoyed.
Play soothing music to provide a sense of comfort.
Based on the person's current abilities you can exercise to music.

Use facial expressions to communicate feelings when involved in these activities.

There are several activities that you can do at home with your loved one. These activities should be simple and do not have to be expensive. According to the stage of your loved one and what you have observed that they can do, you can always find some way of keeping them engaged.

Sometimes just sitting, chatting and singing songs could be one of the best activities of the day at any stage.

<u>Sensory stimulation</u> uses everyday objects to arouse one or more of the five senses (sight, smell, hearing, taste and touch), with the goal of evoking positive feelings.

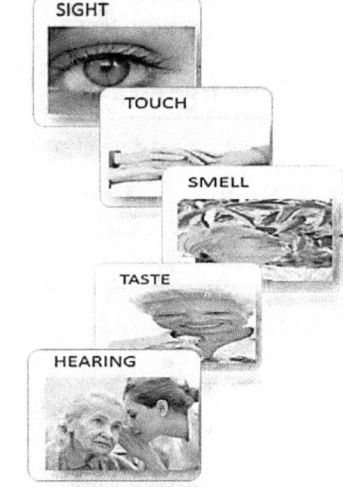

Alzheimer's Tips You Should Know

Ways to stimulate the senses in someone with Alzheimer's Disease

Touch

Massage the person's hands, head, back and shoulders.

Give them manicures and pay attention to hair care.

Hold their hands, play with their fingers sometimes.

Stroke their cheeks gently

Use different textures on the throws, cushions and other materials to stimulate the sense of touch. You may also want to purchase:

Twiddle Muffs

Sensory Activity Aprons

Provide exercise and movement to music.

Alzheimer's Tips You Should Know

Enjoy activities outdoors.

Sight

Take the person outdoors whenever possible. If you are unable to go outdoors then you can watch DVD'S on nature

Stimulate the appetite with the sense of sight by using contrasting colors of food on the person's plate.

Taste

Prepare the person's favorite foods and snacks.

Give them an occasional treat.

Spice up the food with garlic, rosemary, thyme and other herbs. (Do not overdo and see how the person responds, this may not work for everyone.)

Hearing

Alzheimer's Tips You Should Know

Provide music experiences such as dancing, listening, singing, clapping, shaking musical implements and swaying.

Play recorded music or put on TV shows. Avoid too much volume and loud advertisements on commercial radio or TV.

Include them in conversations and be around other family members and friends.

Smell

Be aware of the power of scents and aromas.

Use aromatherapy. **Aromatherapy and Alzheimer's disease**

Use perfumed massage creams and oils.

Be aware of the pleasure of food smells like coffee, fresh herbs and lemon.

"A good deed is never lost: he who sows courtesy reaps friendship; and he who plants kindness gathers love."

Saint Basil

Alzheimer's Proofing Your Home

When Alzheimer's disease enters your family, acceptance will be a major, but important step to take. It will save you a lot of stress and pain in the long run. It is not only acceptance of the diagnosis, but acceptance of changes that have to be made in your life and that of your family. This also holds true for any home where someone with Alzheimer's disease may reside. A home where Alzheimer's is present is usually subject to many changes and adjustments in order to maintain a safe and secure environment for everyone.

If your loved one is living alone, then you will also have to consider making adjustments there, so that they can continue living safely and independently for as long as possible. It is important to understand, that because Alzheimer's disease affects persons differently at each stage, and because changes can occur suddenly, that what may work for one person may only work briefly or not at all for another person. You should therefore make regular observations and assessments of your loved ones condition, to make sure they can continue living alone safely.

Kitchen Safety

The kitchen is one of the most dangerous rooms in your home for the person with Alzheimer's disease. Small appliances, stoves, knives and other gadgets can pose great danger. In this section we offer tips to help you keep your family safe.

Lock away all cleaning products, matches, knives and all sharp edged objects that can harm your loved one or another family member.

Microwaves can be dangerous to the person with Alzheimer's disease

Use flood alarm and anti-flood plug on sinks

Keep electrical appliances from being close to the sink to avoid electrocu-tion if they fall into the sink when plugged

See section on refrigerator

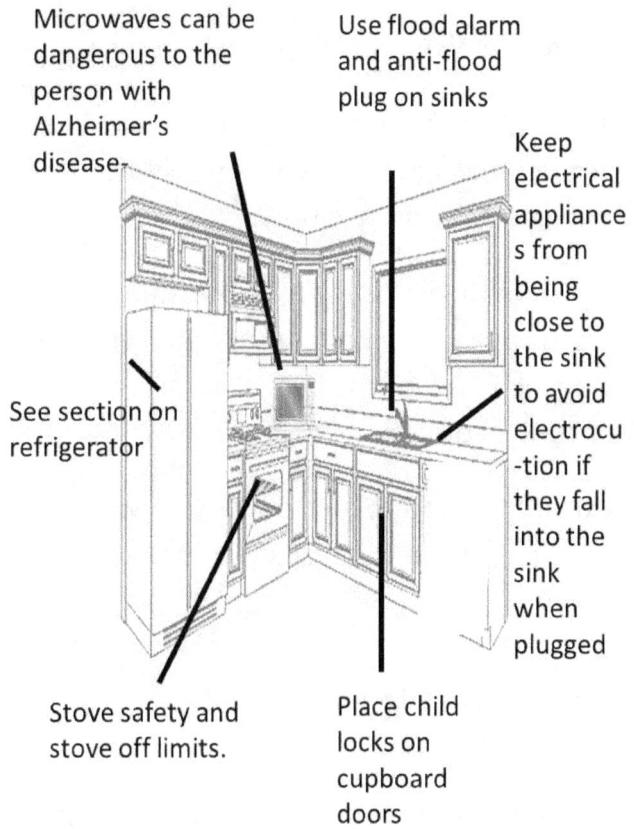

Stove safety and stove off limits.

Place child locks on cupboard doors

Alzheimer's Tips You Should Know

Install childproof door latches on storage cabinets and drawers which have fragile items in them.

Store all medicines in a locked cabinet.

Install safety knobs and an automatic shut off switch on the stove where possible. Alternatively turn the gas off.

Keep decorative artificial fruits and vegetables or anything that may appear edible out of the reach of the person with Alzheimer's disease.

To protect appliances you may need to store them out of the reach of the person.

THE DANGERS OF SMALL APPLIANCES

Small appliances though convenient, can pose great danger for your loved one with

Alzheimer's disease. Prevention is something that should always take priority.

Microwaves can become hazardous because:

The person may cook inappropriate food items such as eggs, in the microwave and they may explode.

They may place aluminum foil or clothes in the microwave.

They may set the time incorrectly and cause a fire.

They can even burn themselves with food or containers that are overheated.

Persons living with Alzheimer's disease tend to pull and fidget at cords, plugs and mostly anything they can put their hands on. They may also place plugged small appliances in the sink with water, this can cause electrocution. **Prevent your loved one from injury by completely removing small appliances from the counter and place them in a cabinet or locked closet.**

Alzheimer's Tips You Should Know

Stoves, Cooking and Refrigerators

Some people in the early and middle stages of Alzheimer's disease may be able to continue cooking on their own. However, because changes in Alzheimer's patients can occur without notice, balancing between safety and independence can be a challenge for caregivers. Allowing a person with Alzheimer's disease to cook on their own must not be left to chance. You should observe carefully on a regular basis, if the person can still prepare their own meals safely. It is not only about safety though, very often persons with Alzheimer's disease just simply forget how to cook and may not be getting the proper nutrition that they need if left on their own. It is possible that they may cook with excessive amounts of oil or salt, cook too much food, eat food that is spoilt and harmful, prepare meats incorrectly or not at all or even put detergents or bleach in the pot.

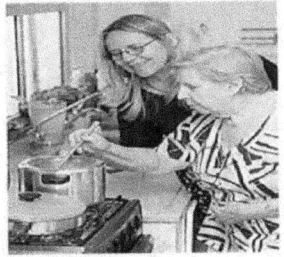 As you monitor and notice increased forgetfulness, you should consider other options for having food prepared.

Stove safety

How to help your loved one with early Alzheimer's disease cook safely

Reminders- Use simple reminders. Place them where the person would see them easily.

Always monitor the person closely and do not depend on the signs.

Use stove turn –off and cooking timers- If the person forgets that they are cooking the timers should turn off the stove automatically (*supervision is still required*)

Use safety burners- these burners will not burn as hot as regular burners do but will

Alzheimer's Tips You Should Know

allow your loved one to boil water and cook a meal. (*supervision is still required*)

Fire Extinguishers- It can be difficult for persons with Alzheimer's disease to operate standard fire extinguishers. There are fire extinguishers that are available that dispense automatically and put out a fire.

Pots, Pans and Potholders –Use easy-to-carry pans with metal that doesn't melt or warp with unbreakable lids and stay cool handles. Use pot holders with flame resistant material and steam and grease barriers which also have bright colors so that they can be easily located. Replace broken pans and pans with wobbly handles.

Stove off-limits

The time will come when the stove must be "off-limits" to the person with Alzheimer's disease. That is why you should always

Alzheimer's Tips You Should Know

monitor the person's ability and the extent of their decline. At this time the person may.

Leave food unattended on the stove

Store flammable items on the stove top e.g. Cloths, newspapers, plastics etc.

They may attempt to cook with plastic containers instead of pots and pans

Leave the gas on or turn on too many burners.

Leave the stove top greasy which may cause a grease fire.

We cannot possibly mention every scenario because there are so many, but the following tips should help you in keeping the stove off limits. You know the person and your situation best so you can choose the solutions that are best suited to you and your family. Sometimes the person may become agitated

Alzheimer's Tips You Should Know

because of limited access, but it is for everyone's safety. Try redirecting their attention to a safer activity.

Remove knobs and store in a safe place- To reduce agitation place a note on the stove where your loved one can see saying "STOVE NOT WORKING"

Use knob covers, but with caution. In some instances the person may be strong enough to pull them off.

Use burner covers but also remove knobs to avoid smoke and fires. Using burner covers may discourage the person from cooking.

Keep matches and lighters out of the person's sight and reach.

Lock the stove if you can. Most new models have locking features for the ovens and in some instances range tops. If you do not have these models then use oven locks that are made to protect children.

Remove fuse- If you only want to have the stove off limit at a certain time of the day you may want to turn off the stove's power temporarily. However, this will not work if you have other appliances connected or if the fuse is located in high risk areas.

Install Remote Switch- You may want to get an electrician to install a separate on/off switch hidden in a nearby kitchen cabinet for your electric stove. If this switch is turned off and your loved one turns the gas knobs on it will not supply power to the oven or burners.

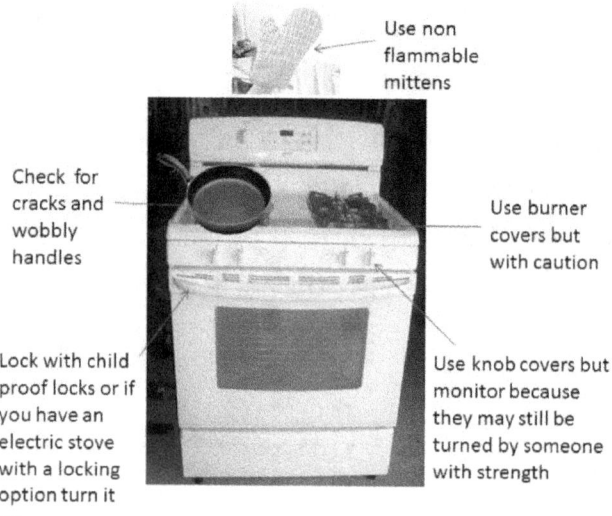

Use non flammable mittens

Check for cracks and wobbly handles

Use burner covers but with caution

Lock with child proof locks or if you have an electric stove with a locking option turn it on

Use knob covers but monitor because they may still be turned by someone with strength

Alzheimer's Tips You Should Know

The refrigerator

As the time progresses, the person with Alzheimer's disease may find it increasingly difficult to determine what items should be stored in the refrigerator. So that, persons especially those living alone, may place meats or other items which require refrigeration in the cupboard or place items for the cupboard in the fridge. With a reduced sense of taste and smell they may not be able to detect spoiled food and may eat what is harmful to them. Some may fiddle with the temperatures, or other parts of the fridge, like the lights or trays or they may leave the door open for long periods.

HERE ARE A FEW TIPS TO HELP YOU:

Regularly visit your loved one living alone and monitor what is happening

Seek assistance from other family members

At times, you may need to put food, medicines and other items under lock and key for the person's safety. However, make this a last resort as some persons may become agitated when they have no-access to the item.

Avoid placing artificial fruit and food decorations on the refrigerator or even on the table as the person with Alzheimer's disease may think they are real and try to eat them.

Your loved one may open the fridge door and forget to close it. Tilting the fridge slightly back and up on the hinge side, will allow it to swing close naturally.

Keep all cords and plugs out of the reach of the person with Alzheimer's disease and ensure that they cannot turn the fridge and other equipment around to fidget with the wiring at the back.

Sinks

Eventually the person with Alzheimer's disease will be unable to perform household chores such as washing and drying dishes and removing food scraps from the sink .Activities that we consider simple will become difficult to manage. So that clogging of the sink is a possibility which in turn may cause flooding. Also the person may forget to turn off the tap when the sink is plugged. To avoid this try the following.

Remove the sink plug and store it in a safe place.

Keep the sink cleared of debris, plates, glasses and utensils or anything that may block the water.

Alzheimer's Tips You Should Know

Use an anti-flood plug which allows a sink to only be filled to a specific level. Once it reaches that level it opens and automatically drains the water to prevent flooding.

Install a flood water and over flow alarm- When water detected can activate music or alarm. The music or alarm will continuously sound until either turned off, removed from water or battery dies

Turn off the water if you will be away for a short period of time.

The Bedroom

When living with someone who has Alzheimer's disease, families and caregivers must understand that the person with the disease sees things differently. As a result, even normal equipment and décor such as mirrors, televisions, and photographs, though they may accentuate the room can be troublesome, as they may cause agitation and fear. Your loved one may perceive people on the television and photographs as real and become upset if they do not respond to them, or maybe, even feel that their own reflection in the mirror is a stranger in the house and cause them to become aggressive and agitated. Different shapes and objects may also appear to be fearful creatures or strangers for persons with Alzheimer's disease.

Tips to keep the bedroom Alzheimer's friendly

A person's own image in the mirror can be mistaken for a stranger and cause them to become agitated. The person may try to remove or fidget with the mirror, it may then become a hazard. REMOVE OR COVER

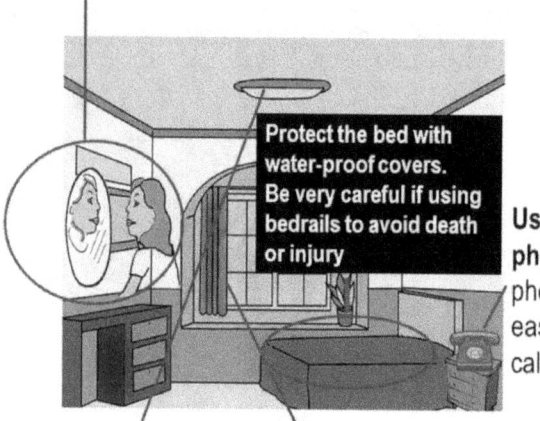

Protect the bed with water-proof covers. Be very careful if using bedrails to avoid death or injury

Use a photo phone for easier calling.

Lighting-The person should avoid bright lights at night. Start dimming the lights shortly before the person goes to bed.

Use blinds to keep out street lights at night or early morning light. Reduce night time agitation for those who perceive reflections of themselves or others as strangers.

Remove or cover mirrors so that the reflection does not frighten the person.

Turn photographs around. In some instances you may have to remove photographs or paintings   altogether as persons with Alzheimer's tend   to fidget or pull at objects in their reach.

Close blinds or drapes early at night. This will reduce hallucinations and the misinterpretation of plants, trees and other objects as things that will harm them.

Increase lighting

Replace patterned furnishings where possible

Remove plants

THE LIVING ROOM

Your living room is your place of relaxation and socializing. You may have it well laid out with beautiful décor, the finest paintings, throw cushions, nice curtains and carpets. However, Alzheimer's disease can change all of that. When living with someone who has the disease, you must be prepared to make adjustments to your home, lifestyle and décor. Safety should become the first priority and that means that some items may have to be changed. In this section you will find tips to show you how to make your living room Alzheimer's friendly.

Never leave person alone with open fireplace

Keep doors closed. Use window and door alarms

Plant pots may be mistaken for the toilet bowl

May be knocked over

Do not leave valuables about , the person may hide them away for safekeeping and forget where they put them.

Throw cushions may be pulled apart by fidgeting and pulling

Use seat protectors in case of leaks

Alzheimer's Tips You Should Know

Page | **78**

Persons with Alzheimer's disease tend to
fidget, and pull at plugs cords and other
objects. Electrical cords can pose a big threat
to them, as pulling these objects apart may
cause electrical shock. Clear them out of their
way and sight of the individual.

Remove scatter or throw rugs and torn
carpets or any objects that may cause tripping
and falls.

Of course your vases, throw cushions and
other decorations accentuate your room, but
if you want to have them around for a long
time it is best to keep them out of the reach
of the person with Alzheimer's disease. (Your
loved one can easily pull apart a throw
cushion, with constant picking and pulling at
the threads)Pulling, picking and fidgeting are
trademarks of some persons living with
Alzheimer's disease.

Place decals at eye level on sliding glass
doors, picture windows, and furniture with
large glass panels to identify the glass pane.

Alzheimer's Tips You Should Know

Do not leave doors open or unlocked as your loved one may easily slip out and wander away.

Use door mat alarms or other simple devices like chimes to alert you of anyone entering or leaving the room

Do not leave the person with Alzheimer's disease alone with an open fire such as a flame on the stove or a fireplace.

Keep matches and cigarette lighters out of their reach.

Persons with Alzheimer's disease may misplace small objects left in their reach, and because of memory loss you may never find them. So keep items such as remote controls, keys for doors or cabinets etc. out of their reach.

Be aware of the fact that your loved one may pull at televisions, radios or DVD players and other equipment that are in their reach. These items can be dragged off shelves onto the floor, be broken and can cause serious injury or fire. Have them mounted or placed higher.

Avoid having the room cluttered. Having pictures and mirrors on the wall and plants in the room, may cause hallucinations, as the person may misinterpret these things, reflections or shadows for strangers in the home.

Have the room well lit for easier vision and close drapes early to reduce shadows.

The Bathroom and Bathing

The bathroom can be a place that has the greatest potential for battles and danger. It is important that it is safe and that the environment encourages your loved one to bathe. While maintaining the style and décor of the bathroom is important, adjustments must be considered to reduce risk for the person with Alzheimer's disease.

Do not leave a person impaired with Alzheimer's disease alone in the bathroom.

Place nonskid mats in the tub or shower to reduce the risks of slippage and falls. Make sure that there are no spills on the bathroom floor that can cause your loved one to fall.

Use raised toilet seats **with handrails**, or install grab bars beside the toilet

Install grab bars in contrasting color to the wall in the shower.

Use a foam rubber faucet cover (like those used for child safety) in the tub to prevent serious injury to the head and other areas in the event of a fall.

To prevent the Alzheimer's patient from locking themselves inside the bathroom it is a good idea to remove the lock on the door.

Do not clutter the bathroom and remove cleaning products and other items that may be hazardous.

If your loved one uses an electrical razor, let him use a mirror outside the bathroom to reduce the risk of electric shock, if he mistakenly brings it in contact with water.

Bathing someone with Alzheimer's disease

Bathing mummy, daddy, husband or wife or any other person who has Alzheimer's disease, can be a daunting task. Along with facing your own personal challenges each day, it is draining to the soul, body and spirit, to try to persuade your loved ones to do what may appear to you to be a simple task. In your mind, it is difficult to understand, why someone who once loved to bathe, no longer sees the need to do so. "I already had a bath" they will tell you, or " where were you when I was bathing?' The individual may use foul language and you may be verbally abused. **Sometimes we cannot change what is happening, but we can change how we respond.**

Remember, your loved one suffering with Alzheimer's is not deliberately trying to hurt you or make your life hell, or make you unhappy. They are simply just not well, and for them bathing can be scary and uncomfortable. Be gentle and respectful, patient and calm.

Prepare yourself mentally and spiritually before you attempt to bathe your loved one. Remember, the key is to remain calm and gentle.

Getting ready for the bath

The supplies

Have everything that you will need for the bath i.e. (soap, towels, clothes etc.) ready and to hand.

Use large towels that will cover the person well and also have washcloths available. Using large towels can help the person retain a sense of privacy which in turn can reduce some aggression.

Use no-rinse shampoo and body wash if you are finding it difficult to give them a water bath or hair wash.

Try not to place the items you need in the reach of the person as retrieving them may be difficult.

BATHROOM SUPPLIES

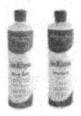 **Shampoo**-If you are washing the person's hair, You may use a no rinse shampoo or mild shampoo to reduce the fear of water coming down on the persons face and irritation of the eyes.

 No Rinse Body Wash or Mild Soap and Moisturiser-. Use mild soap and moisturiser to reduce irritation and for better skin care. No rinse body wash can be used as a waterless bath if you are finding difficulty getting your loved one in the bath.

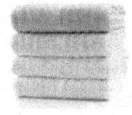 **Towels and wash cloths**-Use large towels for more privacy and washcloths to bathe fragile skin .

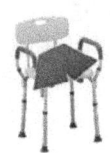 **Shower chair with bright towel**- The shower chair makes bath time safer. Placing a red or bright colored towel on it makes it easier for the person with Alzheimer's disease to see and may reduce fear. You may also use a bright colored shower chair

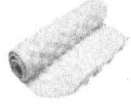 **Non Skid Bath mats**- Prevents slippage and reduces the chances of the person falling.

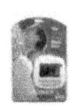 **Bath Thermometer-** Always check water temperature before and during the bath to prevent scalding.

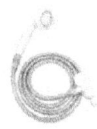 **Hand Held Showers-** Reduces fear of water flowing downwards on the persons scalp and face. Offers greater flexibility

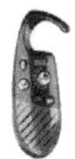 **Waterproof bath radio-** Playing calming music can be soothing to you and your loved one with Alzheimer's disease.

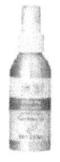 **Lavender Spray-** Keep the room smelling nice with lavender which is known to have a calming effect. Do not over spray

Alzheimer's Tips You Should Know

The room

Remove any objects that may be distractions and cover mirrors. Persons with Alzheimer's disease may not even recognize themselves in a mirror and may think that there is a stranger in the room with them. This can cause fear and agitation and make bathing a challenge.

Check the temperature of the room and warm it up beforehand.

Always test the water temperature before beginning the bath or shower. If the water is too hot or cold it can be a cause of agitation. Severe scalds can occur with water that is extremely hot. If you do not have a thermometer, use the back of your wrist.

Ensure that there are no spills on the floor to cause a fall. A bath mat on the floor by the tub makes the floor warmer to stand on and helps absorb any spills. Use non slip mats or strips in the tub.

Keep the bathroom safe by using a handheld shower head, shower bench, grab bars, and nonskid bath mats. Using handheld showers can reduce the fear of water running down the face of the person with Alzheimer's disease, causing them to be fearful and it also helps in reaching parts of the body easier.

Give the room a nice scent. Research has shown that lavender is useful in reducing agitation in Alzheimer's patients. Do not be excessive.

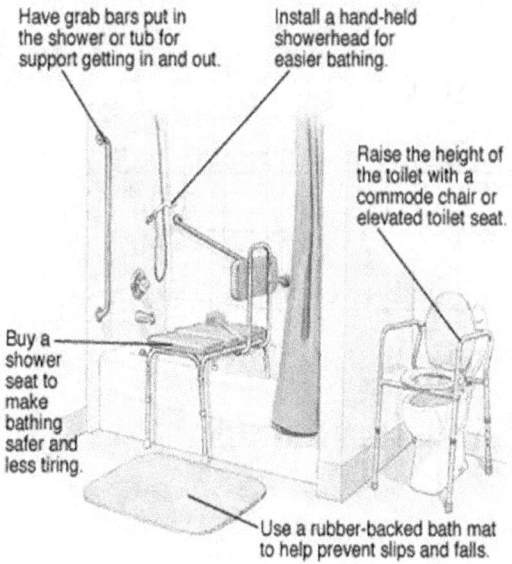

Have grab bars put in the shower or tub for support getting in and out.

Install a hand-held showerhead for easier bathing.

Raise the height of the toilet with a commode chair or elevated toilet seat.

Buy a shower seat to make bathing safer and less tiring.

Use a rubber-backed bath mat to help prevent slips and falls.

Bathroom safety equipment checklist

Shower seat

Rubber-backed bath mats

Grab bars

Hand held showerhead

Commode chair

Raised toilet seat with bars

Preparing "YOU" for the bath

Allow plenty of time so that you do not have to rush the person. A calm attitude and environment reduces agitation and stress, rushing may trigger agitation.

Prepare yourself <u>mentally, spiritually and emotionally.</u> When you approach the person to bathe, be careful to watch your attitude, body language and the tone of your voice.

If you are already angry or overwhelmed by other issues in your life, calm yourself down first before you approach the person.

Many times the aggressive behavior exhibited by Alzheimer's patients is related to fear. Therefore if you are shouting or quarreling, they may also respond in a defiant and abusive manner in an attempt to defend themselves. Shouting, arguing and quarreling will get you nowhere if you really want to see your mum, dad or loved one respond positively.

<u>Coaxing your loved one to bathe</u>

Offer a warm invitation

Say something like "It's time to freshen up" or "Let's get ready to go to church or

Alzheimer's Tips You Should Know

synagogue or temple" (dependent on their faith)

Gently invite them to go out with you, maybe for a walk, to church or somewhere they once enjoyed. Let them know that it's time to get dressed.

Tell them that, a friend or relative or members of the church will be coming to visit and that it is time to get ready. (Please use the name of someone they loved from their long-term memory as they will most likely not remember persons who they met recently.)

Invite them for a tour through the house guiding them gently towards the bathroom, or you can call them to show them something in the bathroom that they like. Once they have entered then you can encourage them to take a shower.

Make yourself smell really nice. Tell them that you want to make them smell just like you and encourage them in.

Try not to say the words bath or bathe in the initial stage of the conversation, this may be a big turn off as they will not think that they need to do any such thing.

Chances are your loved one will resist bathing. What should you do?

When your loved one resists care, step back calmly and think:

Are there any environmental factors such as lighting, shadows, noise, commotion or other external influences that are causing the problem now?

Are there mirrors in the room that may be reflecting images that make your loved one think other people are in the room? Cover mirrors and remove plants or other objects that may cause misinterpretation and hallucinations.

Is it the water coming down on the scalp and face that scares them? Use handheld showers to reduce this problem.

Is your loved one afraid to fall? Reassure them that it is safe and that you will take care of them.

Are there too many people giving instructions at once? Give clear simple instructions.

Are there too many people in the room? Your loved one should still be allowed to maintain their privacy.

One of the questions you will need to ask from time to time, is whether todays confrontation is worth escalating? It is not necessary for your loved one to bathe every day except they are badly soiled. You can use no rinse shampoos and body washes for waterless baths.

If needed, gently take the person's arm and guide him/her into the bathroom.

Alzheimer's Tips You Should Know

If you find that the person is very resistant and a little coaxing isn't working, do another activity and try bathing later. It is amazing how time can change the mood.

How often does the person need to bathe?

It is agreed by many experts that most people do not need a daily bath or shower. Some recommend showering every other day to once a week, while others advise only sponge or bed baths as needed for those easily agitated by showers.

For many individuals, cleaning the face, hands, armpits, and the groin area (especially if the person is incontinent) on a regular basis is what's really necessary. Cleaning the feet is also important, especially in warm weather, to avoid fungal problems and odor.

ALWAYS KEEP THE PERSON'S PRIVATE PARTS CLEAN

Starting the bath

Keep water away from the area of the head and the face to avoid agitation.

Use hand held shower.

Aim at feet and legs.

Give simple instructions step by step.

Be calm and gentle

If your loved one tends to be aggressive giving a favorite snack, wash cloth or finger fidget may have a calming effect.

Encouraging your loved one to help is good for them as it helps them maintain some independence and sense of control.

Give verbal reminders

Show them how

Place soapy washcloth in person's hand

Tell them where to wash e.g Say gently "wash your am"

You can also demonstrate if they do not understand.

Whether you are bathing with a shower or giving a waterless bath it is absolutely important that the person's private areas are clean. This will reduce the risk of infection and is good for the person's overall hygiene. If the person can no longer wash him/herself, then you, someone else or both will need to help them.

Aim hand held shower at feet and legs

Keep water away from the area of the head and the face to avoid agitation.

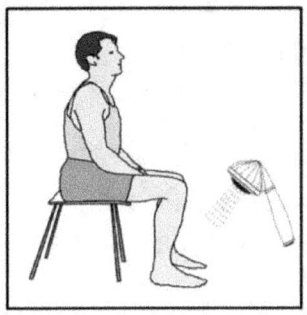 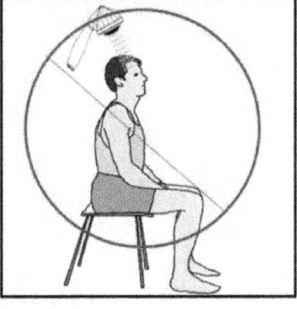

Start by bathing non threatening areas like the back and the arms

Then bathe the private areas

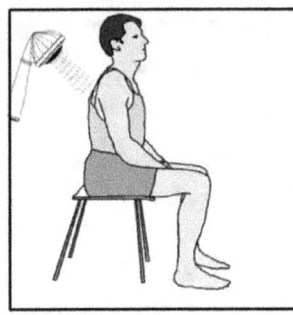 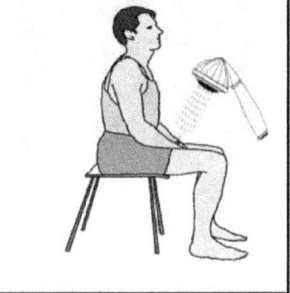

Alzheimer's Tips You Should Know

Dressing and Undressing

Clothing and Dressing

If the person is finding it difficult to choose the right clothing

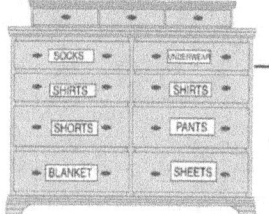 —— De-clutter and Label the drawers

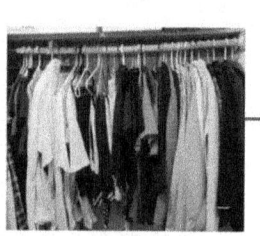 —— De-clutter the closet. Limit choices to avoid confusion. Relocate some of the clothes from the closet

****These suggestions may not work for everyone. Some people may become aggressive and agitated if they think that someone has taken their clothes."*******

Alzheimer's Tips You Should Know

Clothes and Dressing

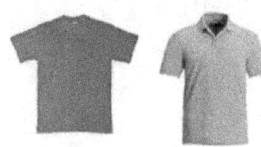

Let them choose.
Ask them
something like: "Would you like to wear your red shirt or blue shirt today?"

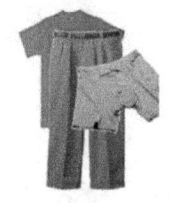

Leave out the clothes to be worn that day in a visible place, in the order which they should be put on e.g underwear on top then pants then shirt.

If the person has difficulty dressing on their own

Choose clothes that are easy to get on and off e.g. pants with elastic waists, blouses with large armholes, velcro enclosures, or large buttons. Avoid clothing with zippers and small buttons as these may be too difficult for the person to handle.

If the person has trouble raising their arms, try special adaptive clothing that open from the back to make sliding them on easier without raising the arms.

Break dressing into simple steps as needed.

Hand the person the clothes item in the order it's to be put on.

Demonstrate the action you want the person to do.

Give simple, step-by-step instructions. For example, "Put your left leg in the pant hole."

Gently show them the arm hole or their arm.

Gently tap the person's leg or arm if they still need assistance.

Don't expect the person to respond immediately Give them plenty of time to dress and repeat instructions if necessary. (Use a pleasant tone of voice.)

Be flexible.
The person may like wearing the same outfit repeatedly, buy duplicates or have similar options available. Always remember that it is important for the individual to maintain good personal hygiene, including wearing clean undergarments, as poor hygiene may lead to urinary tract infections which may further complicate care. Dirty clothes can also affect the social life and your home environment.

If the person wants to wear several layers of clothing don't make a fuss, just make sure that they do not become overheated and that they are dressed appropriately for the weather when outdoors. If clothing is mismatched don't criticize, look for the positive side and offer praise.

If needed lend a helping hand. You may simply start the process and allow the person to continue dressing on his/her own. Sometimes they may only need a little start to remember the process.

A warm smile and lots of praise this can do wonders. However, limit general conversation avoid distraction.

If the person refuses to dress or undress

To help them understand what you want them to do, showing them the clothes you want them to put on may help.

Preserve their privacy. If there are too many people in the room this may cause discomfort. Leave the room with a small opening at the door so you can still observe what the person is doing and intervene when necessary.

The person may insist that there are other people in the room who are not actually there. They may mistake pictures for other people or even their own reflection in the mirror for a stranger. Either remove these or cover them.

If the person remains resistant, stop the activity and direct his/her attention to something pleasant such as a picture of a family member or favorite item. After a period of time, try to resume dressing.

Safety Note

To avoid falls, encourage your care receiver to sit in a chair while dressing, especially when putting on his/her underpants, pants, pullover blouses, socks and shoes.

If the person is constantly undressing

Buy special clothes adaptive clothing that fasten at the back.

The key to remember about Alzheimer's in relationship to clothing is that simplicity will lead to success in getting dressed. If the person can dress independently or with little assistance, select items that have few buttons to contend with, or choose garments with a zipper or the pull on or pull over the head styles. Fewer steps mean the more probability of success for the person with Alzheimer's, especially as the disease progresses and more adaptive, special needs clothing become necessary.

Alzheimer's Tips You Should Know

Make certain that the clothing is washable. Spills, other eating difficulties or incontinence problems will require that clothing be washed on a regular basis.

Please note that some jumpsuits should only be worn if a caregiver is present since the wearer cannot toilet without help.

Places where you can shop for adaptive clothing:

Amazon.com

Silverts

Buck and Buck

Whenever you are confronted with an
opponent. Conquer him with love.

Mahatma Gandhi

Bed Sore Management and Prevention

As Alzheimer's disease progresses, your loved
one may lose their ability to be mobile on
their own. It is very important at this stage to
prevent bed sores which can easily develop if
the person is lying or sitting in one position
for long periods.

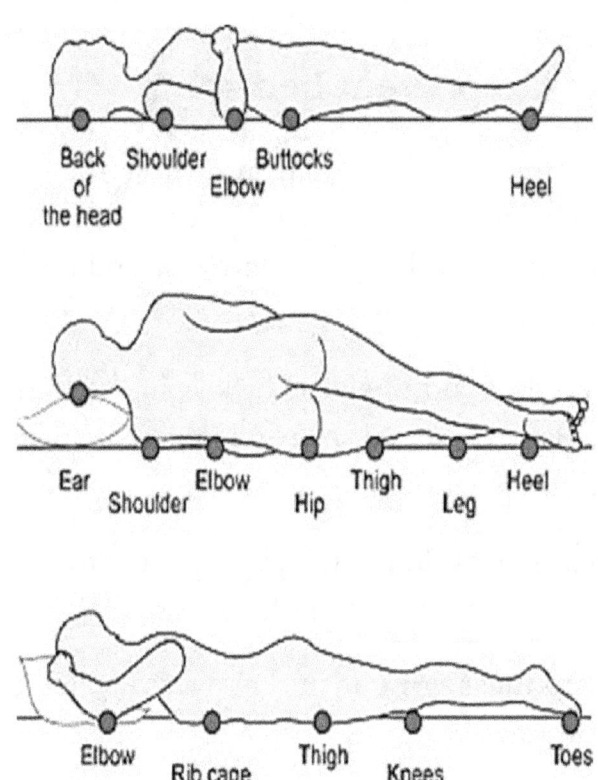

Back of the head — Shoulder — Elbow — Buttocks — Heel

Ear — Shoulder — Elbow — Hip — Thigh — Leg — Heel

Elbow — Rib cage — Thigh — Knees — Toes

FREQUENT AREAS WHERE BED SORES MAY APPEAR

Alzheimer's Tips You Should Know

Tips to prevent bed sores

If you notice a discolored area, check for discomfort, warmness and blanching (whitening) of this area by pressing and then releasing.

Keep their skin healthy by keeping it clean and dry. Use a mild soap and moisturizers so that the skin does not get too dry.

Change wet diapers/clothing often to avoid skin contact with urine.

Avoid massaging their skin over vulnerable bony areas.

Change their body position at least every 2 hours and more frequently if the person is spending a lot of time in a chair.

Alzheimer's Tips You Should Know

Place pillows under their legs from mid-calf to ankle to keep their heels off the bed. **Do not place pillows** under the knees as it can cut off circulation.

Prepare foods with adequate calories, protein, vitamin C and other nutrients, so that the body will be less susceptible to skin breakdown.

Encourage the person to use frequent intakes of fluids throughout the day.

Control blood sugar levels for those with diabetes.

When the person is lying on their back, place a pillow under their lower calves to lift the ankles slightly off the bed.

When the person is sitting in a chair or wheelchair, let them sit upright and straight, as this position will allow easier movement and shifting to help prevent sores.

Use pressure-reducing devices. Egg crate foam mattress pads, gel pads, sheepskin pads, wheelchair cushions, and alternating air mattresses can prevent and minimize the risk of pressure ulcers. Keep in mind that the person should still be repositioned regularly as these devices do not eliminate that need.

"Some days there won't be a song in your heart. Sing anyway."

Emory Austin

Behavioral Management

Managing difficult behaviors in early middle and late stage Alzheimer's disease

WHAT CAUSES DIFFICULT BEHAVIORS?

Moods and behaviors of a person living with Alzheimer's disease can change suddenly and can create worry, stress and frustration for caregivers particularly in the middle to late stages. As the disease progresses the person may become easily agitated angry and abusive, very often for no apparent reason. The person may curse, hurl insults and be verbally abusive. In this section we will look at some tips to help you deal with behavioral problems that your loved one may exhibit.

A person with Alzheimer's disease may lose their ability to communicate verbally because of the changes in their brain. However, they are still conscious emotionally. Always remember Alzheimer's is a disease of the brain not the heart.

Here are a few tips to help you identify what may be causing the problem:

Is your loved one bored?

Try to put yourself in the person's situation. Look at their body language and imagine how they might be feeling and what they might be trying to express.

Assess the situation and see what may have occurred before the behavior. Was it triggered by a conversation, something they saw on television?

Check to see if they may be hungry, cold or maybe need to go to the bathroom

Alzheimer's Tips You Should Know

Does changing the environment help to comfort the person?

How did you react to the problem behavior? Did your reaction help to soothe the patient or did it make the behavior worse?

How to cope with behavioral problems

Caring for a person with Alzheimer's disease is a stressful task which takes a lot of patience, compassion, and love. However, very often the caregiver must remember that they have the ability to create a good and loving atmosphere at home and that their own approach and attitude towards their loved one and the situation, can determine what kind of days you will have together.

Each day can bring a new challenge. It is important that you are in a good emotional state and that you have a good attitude despite the challenges. Ensure that you are calm and at peace with yourself and your own personal situations before you start the day. Putting aside your own personal challenges, whether, emotional, financial or social can be difficult, but it must be done if you are to provide the care, love and support that your loved one needs. If you find yourself becoming anxious or losing control, it is important to take a time out.

Tips to reduce stress

Different stress-reducing techniques work better for some Alzheimer's patients than others, so you may need to experiment to find the ones that best help your loved one.

Exercise is great stress reliever for your loved one with Alzheimer's and you as well. Always consult with your loved one's physician before starting, to ensure that it is o.k. Exercises should be done according to your loved ones ability and the stage of the disease. Walking, gardening, or even dancing are simple exercises that you can do.

Use stage related activities to stimulate and engage the senses of your loved ones; these will also help reduce boredom. For example, finger fidgets, using sensory balls and gel pads, will help reduce boredom, keep your loved ones fingers busy, so that they do not pull at their clothes, and attempt to pull apart the cushions and curtains.

Provide toys that would comfort, such as hot hugs teddy bears.

Aromatherapy is known for reducing stress and creating a calm environment. Research has shown that lavender is the best essential oil to use for Alzheimer's patients.

Simple activities can be a way for the patient to reconnect with their earlier life. Someone who used to enjoy cooking, for example, may still gain pleasure from the simple chore of washing vegetables for dinner. Try to involve the person in as many productive daily activities as possible. Folding laundry, watering plants, or going for a drive in the country can all help to manage stress.

Play calming music or what you know to be the person's favorite music as a way to relax them.

Interacting with other people is still important. While large groups of strangers may only increase stress levels for an Alzheimer's patient, spending time with different people in one-on-one situations can help to increase physical and social activity.

Managing anger and aggressive behavior

As much as you try to create the best environment, there is always the possibility that your loved one will still be stressed, angry, or display aggressive behavior. Here are a few tips to help you deal with this situation.

Watch the tone of your voice, speak quietly, with a soothing voice and be reassuring.

If your loved one becomes aggressive, do not respond in like manner. Remember it is not your loved one, but the disease. Do not take it personally

If your loved one is physically aggressive, back away and ensure your safety.

Always avoid confrontation, remove knives, scissors and any other objects that can be used as weapons out of reach.

Always discuss aggressive behavior with your medical doctor.

If you approach your loved one and you find that they react aggressively, step away for a few minutes or even seconds and come back. Persons with Alzheimer's disease can change moods very quickly and a few minutes can make a big difference.

Hallucinations

Changes in the brain may cause your loved one to hallucinate, that is; having false perceptions of objects or events which involve the senses. The person may see someone in a tree or a chair that is really not there. From time to time you may hear them engaged in a conversation with someone, who you cannot see. Events on television can also contribute to the hallucinations. Here are a few tips to help you with these issues.

Have your loved one examined by their medical doctor, to determine whether medications can help.

Be cautious, monitor the effects that the hallucinations are having, whether they are upsetting or if they are scary. If so reassure them with a calm voice and a gentle touch. Let them know that you are there with them and will care for and protect them.

Do not try to convince the person that what they are seeing or hearing is non-existent. Also remember that the person is not acting or making up stories, but that they are not well.

Try to distract them by suggesting a move to another room.

Try using music or other activities. If the problem is the television, turn it off.

You may need to make changes to the décor or environment.

Reflections or distortions on the furniture or curtains may cause hallucinations. You may need to make changes or turn lights on to reduce shadows.

As the disease progresses your loved one may even lose the ability to recognize themselves in the mirror. When this happens even seeing their own reflections in the mirror can be upsetting, as they may think that it is a stranger or someone wanting to do them harm.

Suspicions

One of the effects of Alzheimer's disease on the individual is suspicion of people around them. As the disease progresses the person becomes confused and there is memory loss. Your loved one may accuse you of "stealing their purse or cutlery" or maybe "trying to hurt them" or a husband or wife may be accused of infidelity. The accusations can be hurtful, but remember that it is not the person, but the disease that is causing these suspicions.

Do not take the accusations personally. Listen carefully to what they are saying and try to understand. Reassure them that you care and that you will assist them with the situation.

Arguing and trying to convince the person that you are innocent, only leads to frustration and stress for everyone. Let the person express themselves and acknowledge their opinion.

Keep any conversations that you will have with the person simple and clear. Offer simple answers.

Try to get your loved one engaged in another activity

Where possible keep duplicates of items which your loved one loses the most.

When being accused by your love one, you may be hurt and be tempted to respond negatively. If you find yourself getting angry, take a time out and consider their plight.

Reassurance, love and compassion are blessings to those whose memories fade.

"One person caring about another represents life's greatest value."

Jim Rohn

Caregivers

Caring for another person is one of the greatest gifts one human can give to another. Families and other persons who commit themselves to the care of people with Alzheimer's disease are indeed special. Alzheimer's disease is a progressive disease, that affects the brain and gradually, every other function of the body. These changes create great challenges, stress, emotional pain and frustration for families, caregivers and care receivers. As caregivers, you must understand the effects that these changes can have on your life and even how you care for your loved one. In this section you will find tips on how to take care of yourself.

Alzheimer's Tips You Should Know

How to take care of yourself

Proper nutrition is very important and eating well balanced meals on a regular schedule is necessary. Take a daily multivitamin. Drink lots of water.

Very often as caregivers we neglect our own needs in order to fulfill those of our care receivers. It is a good idea to prepare your breakfast first in the morning and spend time enjoying a good meal, and then you can get started on your loved one's needs.

Daily exercise such as yoga, gardening, dancing or walking for only 20 minutes will do a lot to keep you fit and in a good frame of mind.

Go outdoors and get some fresh air.

Keep your doctor's appointments and do not ignore your own aches and pains as these may become more serious.

Try to get at least eight hours sleep.

Take time for yourself. Enjoy the things you love, that bring relaxation and peace.

Pay attention to your own emotions and monitor changes that may be negative. Check for signs of depression or stress and get help.

Do not neglect your spiritual needs. Spend time during the day reading inspirational books and magazines. Pray and meditate.

If you are a caregiver to a family member, try not to dwell on the current state of the person, because this can be a very painful experience.

Be thankful that you are there to help and care for the person you love.

Alzheimer's Tips You Should Know

Ask for help. Doing everything your-self deprives someone else of the opportunity to serve.

Do not disconnect from everyone else in your life. Find time for socializing with other friends and family.

Persons, who give care to Alzheimer's patients, go through a lot of emotional and physical stress, which could actually threaten their own happiness and health. As a caregiver taking care of your physical, mental, spiritual and emotional health is a must. If you do not, you may eventually be unable to take care of yourself and also your loved one.

Here are some warning signs that something is going wrong and it is time for intervention:

Withdrawing socially- Do you find that you are having little or no interest in socializing with friends or getting involved in activities you once enjoyed?

Feeling worried – Are you feeling excessively worried about what will happen if you can no longer provide care?

Feeling very anxious-When you think about the future is it making you unusually anxious and fearful?

Depressed-Have you been feeling sad and hopeless for long periods of time?

Indifference – Do you feel like you no longer care about anything that is happening around you?

Tired all the time – Are you always tired, do you feel listless and without enough energy to complete your daily tasks?

Lack of sleep- Are you finding it difficult to sleep or are you waking up in the middle of the night with nightmares?

Extremely emotional – Do you find yourself crying all the time and becoming irritable with the people around you for simple things. Are you shouting and being abusive?

Having difficulty concentrating- Do you have trouble focusing? Are you finding it difficult to complete complex tasks?

Having more health problems- Are you losing or gaining weight, or are you feeling sick more often?

WHAT TO DO

Accept help. Let others help you. Prepare a list of things to be done and let the persons who are willing to help choose a chore. It could be that you can rotate cooking days or even the wash; maybe someone can take the person for walks or do the groceries.

Focus on what you are able to provide. Do not feel guilty, family and friend support is actually one of the greatest defenses for Alzheimer's disease. Accept that you cannot do it all alone, and recognize that it is in the 1best interest of you and your loved one that there are others who are willing to assist.

Get connected. Get in touch with an Alzheimer's association near you and join an Alzheimer's support group where you can meet new friends who are faced with the same challenges as you. This way you can also share your experiences with people who understand the journey.

Seek social support. Make an effort to stay emotionally connected with family and friends. Set aside time each week for socializing, even if it's just a walk with a friend. Whenever possible, make plans that get you out of the house. Many have identified that maintaining a strong support system is the key to managing the stress associated with caregiving.

Set personal health goals. For example, set a goal to find time to be physically active on most days of the week, or set a goal for getting a good night's sleep. It's also crucial to maintain a healthy diet.

See your doctor. Make sure you discuss how you have been feeling and get any test and or medications prescribed.

"The best and most beautiful things in the world cannot be seen or even touched. They must be felt with the heart." – Helen Keller

Communication

The issue of communicating with your loved one will be a matter that families, friends and even staff at care homes will have to deal with at some point. Gradually, as changes in the brain occur, your loved one's ability to speak and communicate will decline. As the disease progresses they will become unresponsive and lose the ability to speak clearly. The sentences may be mumbled and dis-jointed and they will also find it hard to understand what you say. This can be frustrating and emotional for all affected and could last for a long time. This does not mean, that you should stop communicating, or avoid conversations. In this section you will find tips to help you communicate.

Alzheimer's Tips You Should Know

Do not avoid conversations with your loved
ones. Keep talking. Of course their responses
may not be as before, but it helps them
maintain self-esteem and also maintains your
relationship.

Speak normally. Do not make the
conversations complicated. Use simple short
and familiar words. On the other hand, do not
speak "baby talk" .Your loved one is still an
adult and though he may not understand
everything in a sentence. Some words may be
familiar and some they never lose.

In the later stages of my mother's illness,
simple words were what she responded to
best. Words like "Drink" or "Mom" or "come
with me" They were some words that she
never lost like" Thank you". If you keep silent
then how will you know what they know?
Keep talking.

Keep it simple. Give one-step directions.
Ask only one question at a time. Identify

people and things by name, avoiding pronouns.

Their long –term memory is the last to leave .So make conversations a time of memories. Talk about old times, relatives they loved, parents, and grandparents.

Work with them- Your loved one may find it difficult to express themselves clearly. Work with what they give you. So, maybe during the conversation they may mention a name,that could be a talking point. At times the conversation may not seem to make sense for example, they may   say "that they have to go and collect money from someone" Do not argue the point. Continue the conversation and say something like. "O.K I am going to pass by that person, would you like me to collect it for you?"

Never argue. If your name is John and they call you Timothy go along with it or you will spend that time becoming frustrated and stressed out trying to convince them otherwise.

Listen to what your loved one is saying not only verbally but by their body language.

If they call for you, answer and go to them, even though you know they may not even remember what they wanted to say to you.

Gain attention. Gain the listener's attention before you begin talking. Approach the person from the front, identify yourself, and call him or her by name.

Maintain eye contact. Visual communication is very important. Facial expressions and body language are vital ways of communicating. You can tell if a person is frustrated, excited, happy or angry by their body language and facial expression.

Be attentive. Show that you are listening and trying to understand what is being said. Use a gentle and relaxed tone of voice, as well as friendly facial expressions.

When talking, try to keep your hands away from your face. Also, avoid mumbling or talking with food in your mouth. If you smoke, don't talk with a cigarette between your lips.

Be positive. Instead of saying, "Don't do that," say, "Let's try this."

Look for non- verbal cues. Try to understand the words and gestures your loved one is using to communicate. Adapt to his or her way of communicating; don't force your loved one to try to understand your way of communicating.

Facial expression: A **blank or confused** facial expression may signal that there is a problem. A **cringed face** may indicate that the person is experiencing pain of some sort

Ways of talking: the person may have trouble finding words or putting a complete sentence together. This usually occurs in the middle stages of Alzheimer's. Listen carefully for words or names you may recognize. This may help in deciphering what they are trying to say.

Appearance/Attire: Is the person dressed appropriately for the weather? Are clothes matching, or do they look disheveled? Is the person dirty or smelling? These may indicate the progression of Alzheimer's disease to another stage or it could be an indicator that the person may have Alzheimer's disease.

Movements: The person with dementia may have an unbalanced gait or a shuffle. They may have trouble with balance, tripping on uneven pavement or walking around dark places in carpeting. They may make very high and long steps over the lines in tiles. This may happen because of the effects of Alzheimer's disease on vision (these things may appear as holes or larger than they really are)

Actions and Body Movements: Fidgeting, pulling clothes, suddenly jumping up from their seat or bed, roaming and wandering around the house. This could be an indication that they want to use the toilet, or they may be hungry or thirsty and looking for something to eat or they may be bored.

Sounds: Groaning, moaning or grunting may be a sign that the person is experiencing some level of discomfort either physical or emotional. Do not overlook these sounds. Reassure and comfort the person .Ensure that they are comfortable and where necessary consult your doctor

Reduce background noise. Reduce background noise, such as from the TV or radio, when speaking. In addition to making it harder to hear, the TV or radio can compete with you for the listener's attention.

When in conversation with other family members and your loved one is present, try as

Alzheimer's Tips You Should Know

much as possible to **include** them in the conversation. Do not speak about them as though they were not there.

Be patient. Encourage the person to continue to express his or her thoughts, even if he or she is having difficulty. Be careful not to interrupt. Avoid criticizing, correcting, and arguing.

In addition to all of the above, remember that your tone of voice is very important to the conversation. If you are aggressive, agitated or condescending, your loved one will know and it will hurt. Yes, of course they still have feelings. Very often if the care-giver shouts, argues and is aggressive, the care-receiver will respond in like manner. Your loved ones inability to express their feelings normally, does not mean that they are non-existent. A calming voice, a warm smile and a gentle touch will always reach your loved one.

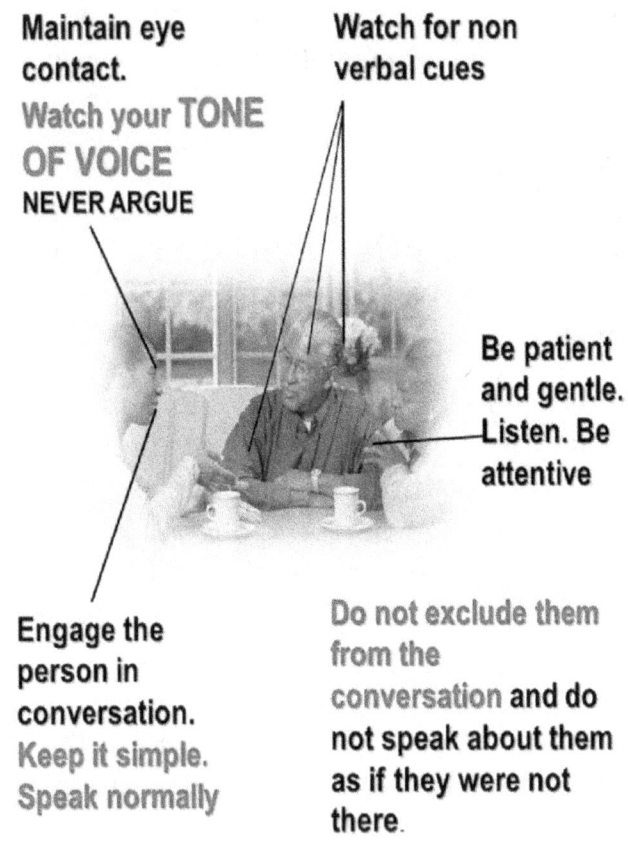

Maintain eye contact.
Watch your TONE OF VOICE
NEVER ARGUE

Watch for non verbal cues

Be patient and gentle.
Listen. Be attentive

Engage the person in conversation.
Keep it simple.
Speak normally

Do not exclude them from the conversation **and do not speak about them as if they were not there.**

Alzheimer's Tips You Should Know

"In the heart of every caregiver is a knowing that we are all connected. As I do for you, I do for me."

<u>Dining Out</u>

Going out to a restaurant with your loved one who has Alzheimer's disease, is a brave decision, and you may be faced with a few challenges. It is a good thing for families to try to maintain a normal life and getting your loved one out of the house is a good idea. In this section there are a few tips for you to consider.

Be selective about the restaurant that you will go to. Is there easy access to facilitate your loved one? Are the toilet facilities disabled friendly? What is the menu like?

Avoid restaurants that are crowded and noisy. Try to arrive earlier than the scheduled time.

Alzheimer's Tips You Should Know

Before leaving home have your loved one use the toilet.

Remember, that as with any outside events, **you should not let your loved one go anywhere alone,** not even to the bathroom.

Consider what stage your loved one is at and their ability to feed themselves. Are they able to use feeding utensils, or would they have to use finger foods.

If your loved one requires special feeding utensils bring them with you.

Depending on the stage of the disease and your loved ones limitations, you may need to **have the meat cut up** before it is served.

Are they going to need a special cup for beverages?

Avoid alcohol and as caregiver, ensure that you are not intoxicated.

When you go to the restaurant, ensure that you are calm and at peace. Remember, that

Alzheimer's Tips You Should Know

your loved **ones mood can change suddenly.** Look out for any indicators that your loved one may be uncomfortable and quickly try to reassure them or if possible remove whatever is causing the problem.

If your loved one is still capable of reading the menu and choosing what they want let them do it.

Persons in the middle or later stages of Alzheimer's, may be unable to order as they may be confused or forget even what they wanted initially. In this case you may have to do the ordering.

Try to avoid buffets. However, if you are at a buffet politely offer to get their meal for them. At buffets there are so many choices of food, that it may confuse you loved one, and cause them to order excess or maybe even create stress for them.

"Caregiving often calls us to lean into love we didn't know possible."
Tia Walker

Mealtime

Understanding Alzheimer's disease at mealtime

Mealtime can be traumatic for the person with Alzheimer's disease, especially in the moderate to late stages of the illness. "Within the framework of their own personality, habits and traits, they are bewildered human beings, bound on all sides by the progressive limitations of their own body and mind, and this is not easy." (Quote from Alzheimer Society of Canada Report, Spring 1982.)

If you have a loved one in the middle or late stages of Alzheimer's disease you may find mealtime to be challenging and sometimes frustrating. It is important to consider though, that because of cognitive decline your loved one's reaction to food and feeding will not be the same. They may see food on their plate, yet fail to understand the connection of their hunger and the food that is on the plate, not knowing that the food is to gratify the hunger or thirst. They may just sit and stare and be unable to start feeding themselves.

This section provides tips and information to make life easier for you and your loved one at mealtime.

Prepare yourself and your loved one

Let the person know that it is mealtime.

Prepare yourself to spend at least one hour with them. Rushing could complicate the whole process.

Expect that you may have to guide the person along the way and that they may be some agitation.

Stay calm.

REDUCE DISTRACTIONS

Turn off the radio and television or put the volume on low.

Put your cell phone on vibrate

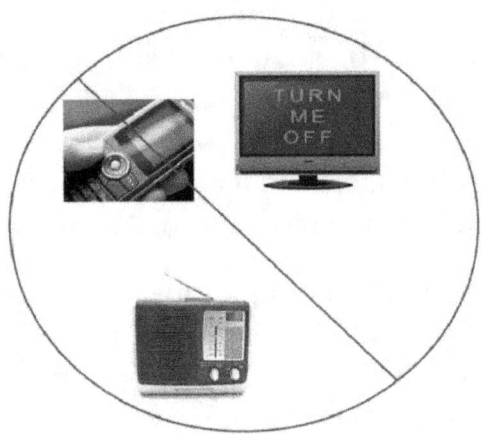

Avoid using patterned plates, tablecloths, or placemats. Patterns can be mistaken for people or animals that are non-existent by the Alzheimer's patient and can create stress and hallucinations.

Simple objects and patterns can create problems for persons with Alzheimer's disease. Even though you may want to continue having your dinner table set nicely, when dealing with a person who has

Alzheimer's Tips You Should Know

Alzheimer's, you may have to make adjustments if you are to cope at mealtime. Your loved one may be confused and distracted by the amount of utensils and cutlery on the table and it could be an interruption to the feeding process.

Serve one food item at a time. One food item at a time, allows your loved one to focus on one action at a time. Your loved one will not be able to maneuver through a plate of food, drink, or dessert, set in front of them all at once. This will distract and create confusion.

Keep the eating area clear of unnecessary items. Unnecessary items on the table are distracting for the person with Alzheimer's disease and you may find them fidgeting, or they may even cause damage to the item or themselves.

**TABLE NICELY SET? MAYBE FOR YOU.
FOR THE PERSON WITH ALZHEIMER'S ITS CHAOTIC**

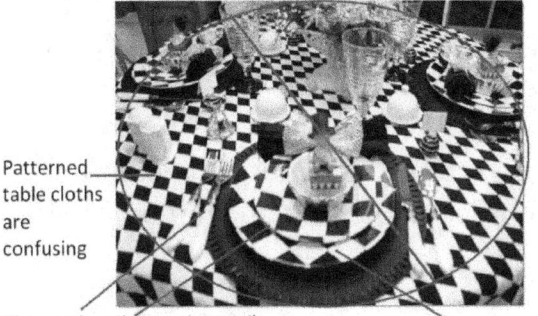

Patterned table cloths are confusing

Too much cutlery and utensils on the table can be difficult to maneuver

Use contrasting plain colored plates and place mats

Make it simple

Keep the table settings simple and clean.

Use soup bowls or another container with sloped sides instead of a regular flat dinner plate. This way the food is not pushed off

Alzheimer's Tips You Should Know

onto the table. You can either use a damp washcloth under the dish to help to hold in place while the food is being placed on a spoon or fork, or purchase a suction plate holder.

Use bowls and placemats that contrast to help your loved one find them more easily.

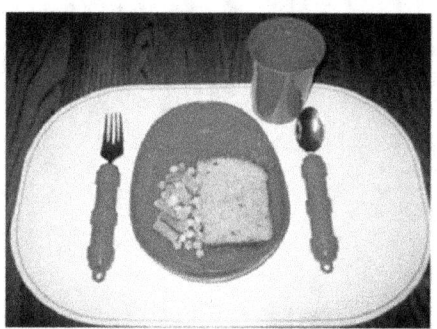

WHY USE RED?

A significant amount of persons with Alzheimer's disease tend to experience weight

Alzheimer's Tips You Should Know

loss. A study out of Boston University suggests that "the weight loss is due in part to the loss of the ability to distinguish contrast between colors. People with Alzheimer's are not able to distinguish light colored food and drink on or in typically light colored tableware. When using tableware that offered a high contrast to the food and drink (i.e.: bright red and bright blue), researchers noticed that the participants in the study increased their food intake by 24% and liquid intake by 84%"

Cups with lids and bendable straws will minimize the number of spills.

Finger foods are probably the easiest to handle.

Chewing difficulties

Slight pressure under the chin or on the lips will start the chewing action

Give simple instructions, "Chew now. Swallow now."

Alzheimer's Tips You Should Know

Remind your loved one how to chew by showing them the proper way to do it

Try to ensure your loved one is comfortable

Feed simple easy to chew meals, stay away from sticky food

Stay away from foods that fall apart or have tough skin

Food that is moistened with gravy, water, or sauce is easier to chew

Cut food into small pieces

Choking on liquids

As the disease progresses, your loved one may find it difficult to swallow food, this can be a testing time for the caregiver as the inability to swallow may cause choking or liquids can enter the lungs and cause pneumonia.

If your loved one is finding it difficult to swallow, **always consult your doctor.**

Alzheimer's Tips You Should Know

Thicken drinks with a tasteless thickener which you can purchase from a pharmacy. Cook cereal with milk or water to help with hydration.

You may also purchase special cups for your loved one which regulate the amounts of liquid to be swallowed at a time by the person.

If your loved one is not eating

If your loved is not eating, you should consider why this might be happening:

Is there an underlying medical problem like an infection?

Is your loved one being left to feed themselves at a stage where they can no longer do so?

Does your loved one need more assistance at mealtime?

Are there too many distractions on the table; is the table setting too complicated?

Are they having problems chewing or swallowing?

Is the food tasteful and stimulating the senses?

What to do

Consult your doctor
Monitor your loved one at mealtime to see what changes need to be made with the table setting and what your loved one is able to handle at this stage.
Add meal replacement shakes to their diet.

Make your loved one's favorite dishes.

Make breakfast or lunch the largest meal of the day.

Ask their doctor about vitamin supplements.

Overeating

If your loved one is overeating consider the following:

Is your loved one bored?

Is the person depressed?

Is food the only means of stimulation?

Memory loss may also be a factor, as your loved one may not remember that they had already eaten.

They may not be able to distinguish between being hungry from being filled.

WHAT TO DO
Consult your doctor.

Alzheimer's Tips You Should Know

Get your loved one engaged in stage appropriate activities as a distraction.

Try having smaller meals 4 times a day.

Make low calorie snacks accessible throughout the day.

Have meals consistently at the same time every day.

Compliment when your love one does well, do not scold if they make an error.

If the person does not open their mouth

Speak to them in simple words say "open" "ahh" "eat"

Place the food on the lips, most times that simple touch gets the eating process going.

Always communicate with your loved one. Never mind which stage they are at. You never know what they will understand. Let them know when it is meal time.

Alzheimer's Tips You Should Know

Guide your loved one through the meal gently, with respectful language and smiles.

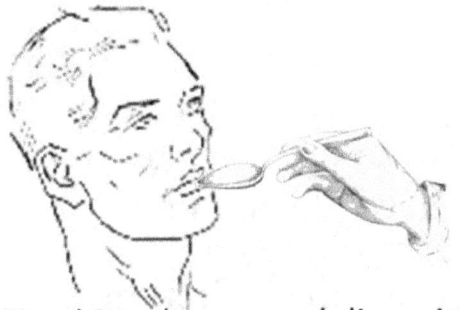

Touching the person's lips with the spoon with a little food or a cup with drink can get the feeding process going and prompt them to open their mouth

Your loved one may start playing with the food. Please remember that they are not being deliberate in this action, they are not being wicked neither are they being nasty. They may simply have forgotten what food is and its

Alzheimer's Tips You Should Know

purpose. Here is where you can help them jump start.

Begin by doing the following:

Sit with them at the table

Say a gentle voice "Pick up your spoon "

Then say "Put some food on your spoon"

Then say"put the spoon in your mouth"

Then say"chew your food"

Then ALWAYS say "swallow."

Alzheimer's Tips You Should Know

If this does not work then you may have to actually start feeding them the first two spoons. Usually they will then get the idea and continue the process.

Encourage them to eat. Don't force them. It's better to say "Have some of this delicious mashed potato" instead of "Why don't you eat your potatoes?"

Say.....

"Have some of this delicious mashed potato" instead of saying "why don't you eat your mashed potato?"

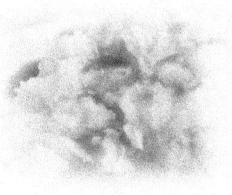

Alzheimer's Tips You Should Know

P a g e | 160

When you realize that your loved one is losing their ability to use the spoon and fork you may be tempted to feed them on your own because it will take a lot of patience to do otherwise.

Resist that temptation. The person should still be encouraged to help themselves in an effort to maintain self-esteem. This may be the time to introduce high nutrition finger foods and drinks. You can also help them to feed themselves. Try these methods.

Drinking using a cup with a handle

It is better to use a cup with a handle for drinking. Very often if the process is initiated the person with Alzheimer's disease will be able to continue the process. However, when your loved one reaches the stage where they are forgetting how to use the fork and spoon, it is also likely that they may also in the middle of eating or drinking forget what they are

Alzheimer's Tips You Should Know

doing. So that if they are left holding the cup or spoon on their own you may have to clean up a lot of spills. You can assist your loved one in feeding themselves by letting them hold the cup by the handle securely, of course this is only if their current abilities allow. Then you can place your hand at the base of the cup and guide it to and from their mouth. That way your loved one is still part of the process as their hand is also involved in the movement to and from the mouth.

1.If current abilities allow, let the person hold the cup by the handle

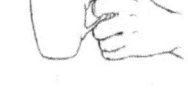

2.Place your hand at the base of the cup

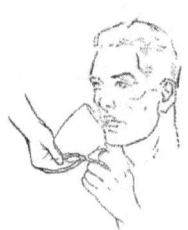

3.Guide the cup to and from the person's mouth and continue this process until the person is finished drinking.

CAUTION: Pay attention to this process as the person may forget that they are drinking and let go of the handle. If the person resist your guidance then you should discontinue the process.

Feeding with a spoon

The same principle applies with assisting your loved one when eating with a spoon. They will be involved in the movement to and from the mouth as if feeding themselves. To begin, gently clasp your loved one's hand as if making a "soul" handshake. With hands clasped into your loved one's hand, place the spoon between your fingers and scoop the

Alzheimer's Tips You Should Know

food from the plate and begin feeding. If your loved one resist this method then you may need to feed them on your own.If you prefer, instead of this method you may also let the person hold the area around your wrist as you feed them. This will also allow them to participate in the feeding process as their hand is part of the movement to and from their mouth.

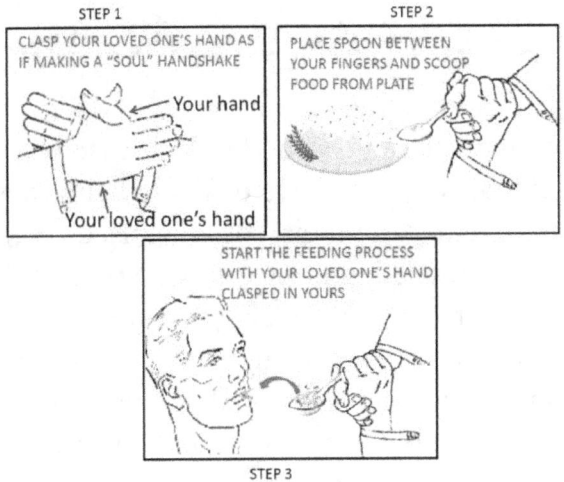

"Fatigue is the common enemy of us all so slow down, rest up, replenish and refill"

Jeffrey R Holland

Travelling with someone who has Alzheimer's disease

If you are thinking about taking a trip with someone who has Alzheimer's disease bear in mind that they may have difficulty with new places, changes in their routine, places that may be crowded and long trips. You should consider this when deciding to take a trip with your loved one. Travelling with a person who is in the early stages is usually better since they may still be able to function quite normally except for some memory loss issues. However, people in the middle or late stages may present a greater challenge as they may have experienced more significant cognitive

Alzheimer's Tips You Should Know

decline and may have lost the ability to understand, reason and carry out regular day to day task.

Travelling by air

Consult your medical doctor to determine whether your loved one is able to travel. Obtain a letter from the doctor explaining your loved ones condition, in the event there are any behavioral problems which may involve security.

Discuss with your doctor the possibility of prescribing medicine that would keep your loved one calm or maybe for travel sickness. Also ensure that you have adequate amounts of the regular medication for the trip.

When making the bookings, alert the airline and hotel that your loved one is memory impaired and about any special arrangements and precautions that should be considered.

Avoid long trips and fly nonstop. If they are any delays, try to find a place that is comfortable, not too crowded or noisy to wait.

Always have a plan B, in case a flight gets cancelled or if any unexpected events occur.

When booking, ensure that you get a seat side by side

Pack early, check and recheck that you have all the necessary documents, medication, incontinence products etc.

Remember you must keep your loved one close to you at all times. Do not take excessive luggage that would require the use of both hands. One hand should be free for your loved one to prevent them from wandering.

Make sure you have all important documents near at hand and place any small items that may set off the metal detector in a zip-loc plastic bag and place them in your carry-on bag.

Do not allow your loved one to carry anything important, they may lose them or forget where they are.

Take along games that will keep your loved one busy and ensure that there are plenty of snacks and drink and a blanket and pillow for comfort.

Travelling by car

When planning a trip with your loved one who has Alzheimer's disease, it is better to take short trips. Long trips by car are not a good idea, particularly if it is only you and your loved one.

This section outlines some tips to consider when taking a car trip with a person living with Alzheimer's disease.

It is always a good idea to travel with other persons who can drive.

If your loved one appears agitated or aggressive, you should not take the trip alone. This can pose a danger to you and other road users.

If during the journey your loved one is agitated, or needs attention stop at the first available place. Never attempt to give assistance or calm him down while driving.

Keep car doors locked, and seat belts on, if you can, activate the child locks.

Bring along activities suitable for Alzheimer's patients, that can be used in the car like sensory balls, hot hugs teddies, or finger fidgets which can keep your loved one busy.

Play your loved one's favorite music and sing-a-long.

Plan stops for rest regularly and remember to never leave your love one alone. Stick to them like glue. Wandering is always a possibility with persons having Alzheimer's disease.

When you arrive at your destination do not forget that your travelling partner has Alzheimer's and therefore the same hygienic requirements and safety precautions such as, checks **for water temperature in the baths, reducing the risk of falls**, etc. should apply.

"Impossible situations can become
possible miracles."

Robert H. Schuller

Wandering

Research shows that six in 10 people with
Alzheimer's and other dementia will wander.
Unfortunately some of these persons never
return alive. The person may become
disoriented and confused and without
intervention may wander somewhere that they
cannot be helped and die. It is very important
therefore that families and caregivers always
place high priority on safety and wandering
prevention.

Who is at risk of wandering?

As long as your loved one has memory loss
and is still able to walk, there is the potential
for wandering. Even in the early stages, a
person may wander and become confused.
Families should consistently monitor loved
ones who have been diagnosed with

Alzheimer's Tips You Should Know

Alzheimer's disease as wandering can occur at any time. A regular trip to the store next door may end up leaving you and your family with a heart ache.

Always look out for warning signs even if there has been no diagnosis of Alzheimer's or other dementia.

You may notice your loved one preparing to go to work when he has already retired.

Packing bags with clothes, is restless and pacing the room particularly at sun down.

Insisting that they need to "go home" when they are already at home.

Returning home later than usual from shopping or other familiar trips.

Finding difficulty locating familiar places like the bathroom, bedroom or dining room.

Trying to locate current or past friends and family and asking about them often, even the deceased.

Alzheimer's Tips You Should Know

Acting as if they are doing a hobby or chore, but nothing gets done

Appears lost in a new or changed environment

Tips to prevent wandering

Remember that no strategy is fail proof and wandering may still occur no matter how diligent you are. In this section you will find some tips to help reduce the chances of your loved one wandering.

Monitor the time when your loved one becomes restless

Plan stage appropriate activities around the time that they become restless and want to "go home" Activities and exercise can reduce anxiety, agitation and restlessness.

If your loved one insist on "going home". Do not shout or argue or try to persuade them that they are already there. Talk with them as if they are right. In a calm voice,

Alzheimer's Tips You Should Know

reassure them that they are safe and that you will be going home soon after you have finished a task.

If for some reason your loved one becomes very aggressive and you cannot keep them at home. Make sure that you walk with them and call for help. After some time of walking, you can then say something like "Mom, let's go home now" very often they will go with you willingly.

Ensure that the basic needs of your loved one are met, for example that they are not hungry or thirsty and therefore feel the need to go in search of food.

Avoid places that are busy and confusing and that can cause disorientation. For example: shopping malls, or grocery stores.

Purchase window **and door alarms** or other devices that will signal if someone is exiting the house. Simple things such as bells or chimes which are loud enough can be used also.

Alzheimer's Tips You Should Know

Never lock the person with dementia in at home alone, or leave them in a car without supervision.

Do not leave your loved one at home alone. If you are travelling, walking, gardening, shopping or engaged in any outdoor activities make sure you stick to them like glue.

Be careful not to leave doors open even if you are only in the other room.

Keep car keys out of sight and reach. A person with dementia may drive off and be at risk of potential harm to themselves or others.

Use electronic devices **such as GPS trackers** that can assist in locating the person if they go missing. Also let them wear jewelry I.D.

Involve your neighbors and friends by asking them to call if they notice your loved one anywhere alone.

Notify the police immediately if you discover that your loved one is missing.

Prepare an identification kit today.

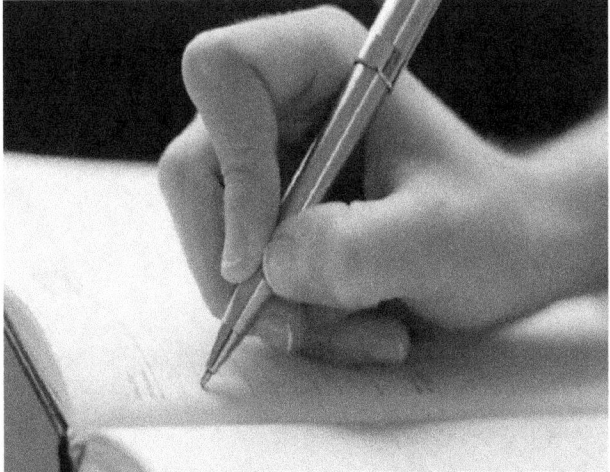

This is very important in the event that your loved one gets lost. This kit should include vital information such as their basic information e.g name, address and date of birth; physical description e.g. height, eye color, hair color etc.; identifying features such

Alzheimer's Tips You Should Know

as scars, tattoos etc; a recent photo and medical information. Keep this information in a location where you can easily access it.

"When you think you've reached the end of your rope, tie a knot and hang on"

Thomas Jefferson

DEALING WITH THE MESSY ISSUES

TOILETING AND INCONTINENCE

Toileting and incontinence are personal and private issues that can eventually create nightmares for caregivers of persons with Alzheimer's disease.

As the disease progresses and your loved one reaches the middle and later stages, they may experience urinary or fecal incontinence. This can be a very traumatic time for your loved one and also a time of extreme challenges for you. As a result of their cognitive decline and their inability to reason, understand and interpret, they may also engage in dysfunctional behaviors feel like they would

Alzheimer's Tips You Should Know

drive you crazy. Coping with behaviors like peeing in the plant pots, playing with feces and smearing it on the walls, even sometimes putting it in their mouth are painful and difficult to handle .

In this section you will find tips and ideas to assist you in coping with these messy issues whilst helping to maintain your loved one's dignity.

WHAT IS INCONTINENCE?

Incontinence is the inability to control one's bladder and /or bowel elimination. Usually in persons with Alzheimer disease bladder incontinence is experienced before bowel incontinence.

WHAT IS URINARY INCONTINENCE

Urinary incontinence is the loss of bladder control resulting in the involuntary loss of urine. The severity of urinary incontinence can range from the occasional leaking of urine

Alzheimer's Tips You Should Know

when you cough or sneeze to having a strong and sudden urge to urinate but you cannot get to the bathroom on time.

Incontinence can be a very embarrassing problem for anyone and even though your loved one may have lost some of their ability to think and function, they may still continue to feel ashamed and humiliated at this stage. It is important therefore, that you be gentle, compassionate and supportive when your loved one reaches this phase.

WHAT MAY CAUSE URINARY INCONTINENCE

A decline in the person's intellect and loss of memory very often interferes with the person's ability to think and intellectualized what is happening around them. In the late stages incontinence becomes not only a matter of the person's inability to think but also the body's inability to function normally.

Alzheimer's Tips You Should Know

At this stage your loved may have lost total control of both and simply urinates involuntarily.

WHAT IS FECAL or BOWEL INCONTINENCE

Fecal incontinence also known as bowel incontinence incontinence, is the inability of the person to control bowel movements. In the late stages of the disease you may find that the person may uncontrollably leak stool from the rectum. The severity can range from passing small amounts to a total loss of bowel control with bowel movements occurring at any time or several times throughout the day.

SIGNS OF INCONTINENCE

Your loved one may sit in one position for a long time to avoid embarrassment.

You may smell urine or fecal odors about the house.

Alzheimer's Tips You Should Know

When your loved one gets up from sitting and walks you may see a trail of urine.

You may find that the chairs, bed or clothing of your loved one are soiled or wet.

WHAT TO DO IF YOU NOTICE URINARY OR FECAL INCONTINENCE

If you notice any signs of fecal or urinary incontinence in your loved one you should:

Consult your doctor to determine if the cause of incontinence may be related to a medical condition other than Alzheimer's disease such as urinary tract infections or prostrate problems.

Consider the use of adult diapers and other incontinence products such as seat protectors, bed pads and underpads.

Look for signals which may indicate that the person may want to go to the bathroom. Fidgeting, pacing up and down the room, getting up from the bed or chair, or even pulling at their clothes.

In the early and middle stage the person may still be able to find the bathroom on their own. **Place clear signs and directions** to make the bathroom easy to find. Keep the door open so that the toilet is visible.

Keep the bathroom safe. (Read chapter on Alzheimer's proofing your home   Bathroom Safety)Ensure that there is proper lighting in the bathroom.

Remind the person to use the washroom, especially after meals and before bed. Do this in a gentle and sensitive manner.

Adaptive clothing that makes it easy for undressing and dressing are ideal for these situations. For example, clothing with elastic waist instead of a button or zipper.

Alzheimer's Tips You Should Know

Use commodes, urinals, incontinence briefs, under pads and other supplies for daily living

Consider changing the color of the toilet seat. A red seat paired with a white toilet bowl may be easier for the person to see.

GETTING OVER THE STIGMA OF WEARING ADULT DIAPERS.

Even though incontinence is a condition that affects millions of adults with and without Alzheimer's disease, for many there is still an embarrassing stigma attached to it. As a result, some people are ashamed to even shop for adult diapers and other incontinence aids for fear that others may feel that they cannot control their bladder or bowels. Sometimes persons with Alzheimer's disease may resist wearing these diapers, because they may not have accepted the fact that they need help or because they may feel that wearing diapers are demeaning and for children. On the other hand for the family caregiver, having to accept that their loved one needs to wear adult diapers can also be a difficult thing. However, adult diapers can save you and your loved one a lot of embarrassing moments, reduce the amount of cleaning you have to do, allow you and your loved one to be active rather than hiding away at home for fear of spills and generally can reduce the stress and frustration that can be associated with incontinence. The diapers are usually undetectable and in many ways help to maintain your loved one's dignity.

Attitude and Adult diapers (click here)

Here are a few tips to help:

Accept that your loved one's abilities are changing and what they need is help with a situation that they cannot control. Get over your own pride and misconception about the issue.

Be empathetic and discuss the need with your loved one, explaining that they are only being used in case there is an "accident". Show them how they can help.

You may want to involve the doctor in the process of suggesting that they wear the garments. They may be able to influence your loved one more.

Avoid using the word diaper; your loved one may recognize the word and some persons may find it demeaning.

Alzheimer's Tips You Should Know

Use a diaper that looks more like the regular undergarment such as pull ups, Take the steps to purchase the right size. You may not get it right initially but eventually you will find the best fit.

How to choose the correct diaper (click here)

Do not get angry if your loved one resist, try discussing the matter at a later date but keep at it.

If your loved one is at a stage where you assist them in dressing, fit the diaper into the panty or regular brief and pull them on at the same time.

Continue the use of their regular undergarments with the diaper.

FEAR & EMBARRASSMENT = AGGRESSION

If the time comes when using adult diapers cannot be avoided, your loved one will need all the support they can get. This may perhaps be the most important thing for you to remember at this stage.

Your loved one is very likely to feel fearful, embarrassed and out of control when incontinence begins and may at times become aggressive when you attempt to intervene. Try to understand what they are going through and be gentle, calm and compassionate. This is the time that they need you as they battle with the effects of Alzheimer's disease. Do not humiliate or insult them if they have soiled their clothing or your favorite chair.

Even though it is also an agonizing and painful process for you, do your best to make life easier for them.

PEE IN THE PLANT POT

Many families and caregivers have experienced the shock of smelling urine or stool in the house but not knowing why or where exactly it is located. Some may have actually caught their loved ones peeing in the plant pot, in cups, in the sink, on the bed or under the pillow or virtually anywhere in the home. This is one of the behaviors that give families and caregivers the biggest shocks and challenges within the home. Finding a way to stop your loved one from peeing or having bowel movements in inappropriate places can give you headaches. It requires compassion, tolerance an enormous amount of patience, a good stomach and sometimes a little humor. The reality is that these are messy issues and sometimes your loved one may also exhibit aggressive behavior making it double trouble to clean.

In order to survive the challenges that you may face with this issue you should first consider what is happening to your loved one. You awareness of the difficulties your loved one is facing will change any distorted perspective you may have as to why they are doing these things. Your loved one is definitely not trying to make you unhappy; neither are they attempting to destroy your home. They are also not being evil or wicked.

WHY?

Always remember that your loved one is gradually losing control of their mental and physical abilities because of damage to the brain. All the social norms, training and behaviors which were instilled from a child are gradually fading. Their ability to connect their urges to urinate or stool with going to the toilet will progressively erode and even though they may still remember that they need to go, they may find difficulty in deciphering where. So can you see why they would choose to pee in the plant pot or the bath tub or sink? The shape is somewhat similar to that of the toilet bowl. To you it is just a plant pot however, for the person with Alzheimer's disease it is the toilet bowl. In some cases they may just know that they need to go and ease themselves anywhere.

Here are a few things to consider if your loved one is peeing and stooling anywhere:

Your loved one may find it difficult to locate the washroom.

They may find it difficult to undress.

Their inability to communicate their need to go to the toilet can cause some persons to soil themselves.

It may be that they may simply forget to use the toilet, or how to do so.

Your loved one may not understand and or be able to interpret the bodily sensations which indicate that it is time to use the toilet.

There are several steps involved in using the toilet (locating the bathroom, undressing, using toilet paper, etc.) as dementia progresses; it can become increasingly

Alzheimer's Tips You Should Know

complicated for the person to carry out a series of steps.

They may find it difficult to distinguish the difference between the toilet bowl and other similarly shaped items in the house.

WHAT TO DO

You may have to make some adjustments to the décor in your home. Where necessary and keep plant pots, tubs etc. out of their reach.

Place clear and simple signage on the bathroom door.

Use anti-strip clothing that makes it difficult for the person to undress at will.

Schedule a time for them to use the toilet routinely.

Items that look similar to the toilet bowl that cannot be removed should be covered.

Monitor the person and look for signs that they may want to use the toilet, e.g. pulling at clothes, being gittery and looking around for something.

Listen to what they are saying, they may be trying to signal to you that they want to go to the toilet but may say something else.

FECES- PLAYING AND SMEARING

One of the least talked about behaviors in persons with Alzheimer's disease is the playing with or smearing of feces. For some it is an embarrassing and private issue that they would rather not let anyone know about for fear of scorn and rejection. However, this behavior is quite prevalent in persons who have Alzheimer's disease and many families and caregivers find it very difficult to cope with.

As your loved one continues to experience cognitive decline, they may start playing with their feces and sometimes smear it on the walls, wipe it in the curtains, on their face, sometimes they may even throw it at you or put it in their mouth.

Why is this happening? Are they just being totally disgusting and deliberate in their actions? The answer to those questions is **NO!**

The tasks of cleaning feces from the walls, carpet, chairs, other areas of your home and your loved one's body can drive you to tears. It is not a pleasant job by any means and the fact that after all the cleaning the day before you may have to do it all over again the next day is not stressful. Fortunately, there are some steps that you can take to lessen the impact of your loved one smearing and playing with their own feces.

Limit access. If the person is unable to touch their feces, then you will have no playing or smearing. Use adaptable clothing that are available in both day wear or sleepwear such as anti- strip suits and jumpsuits that restrict the person's ability to undress themselves and to dig into the diaper or anus. If these are not available try leotards that reach just above the knee that they can wear under regular clothing. Ensure that the clothing is always comfortable and clean.

Clean stool quickly, whether it is in the diaper, on the floor, bed or wherever.

Monitor the person when they go to the toilet, they may forget how to wipe or may see the stool in the toilet bowl remove it, attempt to throw it away and end up splattering the walls.

In some cases your loved one may find the toilet easily but when they get there, they may be unable to decipher where exactly the toilet bowl is and may stool on the floor, the bath tub, waste basket or anywhere they think is the toilet. To assist with this problem, you may contrast the color of the toilet seat so that they can clearly identify where to go. For example: If your toilet bowl is white, it is recommended that you use a brighter color like yellow or red. Red seems to be the color that stands out for persons with Alzheimer's disease but any contrasting color would be helpful.

Monitor the person's behavior for signs of irritation or an infection that may be causing them to itch in the anal or vaginal area. If this is true, the person may be scratching the area for relief and may inadvertently get feces on their hands. In an attempt to get it off they may wipe or smear it on anything in sight. This could also happen if the incontinence garment is uncomfortable, not fitting well or is itself causing irritation. Consult the doctor immediately if you suspect that the above-mentioned may be happening.

Frequently monitor your loved one in order to reduce the possibility of them stooling without your knowledge and smearing it everywhere.

Do not isolate them in their room even when you have visitors this provides the perfect opportunity for them to strip and meddle. Keep them in your view so that you can intervene if they attempt to do so.

HOW TO HANDLE THAT DREADED CLEANING UP

We all have our own ideas and draw backs about feces. A lot of those ideas are determined by whose feces we are cleaning. A parent or adult usually has no problem cleaning the stool of a child if they get messy, however, there is a fear attached to cleaning an adult. For children who now have to carry out that same task for their parents, there is also the emotional pain of role reversal and watching the demise of a loved one who can no longer care for their toileting needs. Some people cannot bear the thought that they have to clean their mummy or daddy; they feel uncomfortable bathing and cleaning the intimate and private areas of their parent's body. Others see feces as an awful and dreaded thing and they will not go near it for any one or any reason.

Whether your loved one has defecated in the waste basket, on the carpet, or chair, your attitude is the key to how you will cope and clean up. Your attitude and perception of the situation that you face will determine how difficult the tasks ahead will be. The most valuable tip you will find in dealing with this issue, is the one that recommends a change in attitude and perception. It will make cleaning less frustrating, less frightening and will help in keeping your gut down.

Accept it for what it is. Feces is waste matter that comes from ingested food , which is rejected by the body mixed with secretions from the intestines and having a bowel movement is an essential function of the body. Yes, there are unpleasant odors associated with it; this is so for any kind of feces whether it is dog, cat, child or adult and it can be unhygienic to touch. There is nothing mysterious about it; neither will it explode on you if you get too close.

Taking the first step- The very first time you have to clean stool is always the most difficult, you may find yourself wanting to throw up because of the smell and your perception about stool. However, if you do it once, then the other times become less difficult. The truth is that the more you it, the less frightening and intimidating it becomes. Eventually even the odor will have less effect.

11 SIMPLE THINGS YOU CAN DO TO MAKE CLEANING A WHOLE LOT EASIER.

Cleaning feces from the person's body, walls and sheets can be made a lot easier with these few tips.

Reduce the unpleasant smell by using disposable anti- odor face mask, using regular masks and placing a drop of your favorite scented oil on it or even placing skin sensitive oil with a fragrance you love on your upper lip.

<u>Use a hand held shower</u> that makes reaching the difficult areas of the body easier when showering.

If you are finding it difficult to get the person in the shower or to wash their hair, use no rinse shampoos, body washes or perennial skin cleansers that are no rinse.

Learn to breathe differently. Try not to take deep breaths in, instead breathe out for longer periods and in shorter puffs or practice holding your breath for longer periods.

Move quickly. Don't fool around, get straight to the task, baggage any soiled diapers quickly and wash soiled clothing immediately.

<u>Always use disposable gloves</u> as protection whenever you are cleaning stool or washing soiled clothing.

If you use a<u> commode</u> it is a good idea to use commode liners to help with the easy and hygienic clean- up of the commodes.

Protect beds and furniture with **<u>seat protectors</u>**, **<u>sheet protectors</u>** and **<u>mattress covers.</u>**

Always have a ready supply of your preferred cleaners available. You will never be certain when an incident will occur and there really will be no time to go shopping when it happens.

Make it a priority to keep the person's nails short. Trying to clean feces from underneath fingernails can be difficult and frustrating, especially if the person is not co-operating.

Alzheimer's Tips You Should Know

Be compassionate. No doubt coping with incidents of smearing and playing with stool and having to change soiled diapers and clothing are never easy. There are times when you may be tempted to scream or shout at the individual and even think that they are doing it deliberately. As difficult as it may seem for you try taking a walk in your loved one's shoes, where they are losing their ability to reason and think and they have no control over their bodily functions. Think of having to depend on someone to clean and wipe them because they can no longer do so themselves and imagine the fear and trepidation they may feel having lost control and being shouted at and insulted. Your loved one may lose many things, but they still understand aggressive behavior towards them, they understand by your facial expressions and when you are angry. Likewise they also can sense the compassion and love you extend through a gentle touch and a warm smile. Even though it is challenging try you best to be compassionate.

Alzheimer's Tips You Should Know

"When you think you have reached the end of your rope, tie a knot and hang on."

Thomas Jefferson

The Spitting Dilemna

Many people with Alzheimer's disease go through the early, middle or late stages of the disease. However, not everyone faces the same challenges at the same time and some people may exhibit behaviors that are different to others. In the middle stages you will start to see more significant decline, forgetfulness, unusual changes in moods and behavior, incontinence issues and general changes in their ability to function as normal. As the disease progresses to the late stages, your loved ones ability to communicate verbally, reason and understand would have almost been lost along with other, functions.

During these stages, there can be some shocking and alarming behaviors that become

Alzheimer's Tips You Should Know

a part of their struggle with the disease. One of these is spitting.

The person may all of a sudden start accumulating saliva in their mouth for a long period, and then spit it out anywhere, on anything or anyone.

This is very trying period for families and caregivers and can become a nightmare. It creates a social, hygienic and emotional dilemma for everyone involved.

SOCIAL DILEMNA

The spitting problem is one that is destined to create social problems for families. When your loved one is at the stage where they spit indiscriminately, it is difficult to take them out of the home to shop, to a restaurant or even to church for fear that they may spit on someone. It may also affect how you socialize within the home, whether or not family members feel comfortable inviting people to their home and if they do, will the person with the disease be kept in isolation? In some

Alzheimer's Tips You Should Know

cases, some friends and family may avoid coming to the home and may scorn you and your loved one. Some members of the household may react patiently, others may become very irritated by the spitting and this may cause a strain in relationships. It also limits your options for help in caring for the individual, because whereas you may understand and try to cope with the situation, other people just will not make that sacrifice. The reality is that where there is uncontrollable spitting by your loved one, there will be anxiety and the fear about having people around or taking your loved one outside of the home because generally people see spitting as a social indignation. You also would not want them spitting on others because that is unlawful and can even though the person may not have been spat on deliberately.

HEALTH HAZARD

It is well documented that saliva hosts a variety of diseases and infections. Apart from the fact that it is risky to socialize with someone who spits everywhere indiscriminately, it is also a health hazard in and out of the home. We all know the slogan" spitting spreads diseases" and so your concern about your loved one's spitting problem is justified. Viruses such as the flu, colds and such like could be easily spread as a result of this seemingly uncontrollable problem.

EMOTIONAL AND MENTAL STRESSOR

You have asked him time and time again, to stop spitting, actually you have done more than ask, you have begged. However, all your begging goes on deaf ears, a few minutes after, there goes another mouth full of spit on the curtains or carpet. How stressful and distressing. You may have tried giving them a cup to spit in, tissue and showing them the sink but nothing works. You have to constantly walk behind them and clean up, or try to locate the last set of spit which you missed. This helpless situation has you at your wits end.

WHO IS IN CONTROL

I understand what it is like to be mopping every minute, constantly cleaning walls and windows, or following to see where the next set of spit is going. Chances are that if you have picked up this book, either you, or someone you know might be facing the same issues.

In this situation all the odds seem to be against you. You are unable to get your loved one to do what you want. Your social life is being changed. Your home has been invaded by a spitting frenzy, with carpet, furniture, curtains, the floor, the walls everything being doused in spit. This is a very trying time, and you feel helpless and out of control. Are you really?

As you attempt to deal with the spitting dilemma, I want you to place in the forefront of your mind that you are indeed the person in control of this situation and that you are the one who can make a change. After all you are the person who still has the ability to understand reason and determine what appropriate or inappropriate behavior is. You still have the ability to control your moods, to verbally communicate what you are feeling and to remember what you just did. The reality is that though you are facing a difficult situation day by day, you are still the one who holds the key to a solution.

WHO IS NOT IN CONTROL

Alzheimer's disease is a brain disease that slowly destroys memory and eventually the ability to carry out the simplest tasks. It begins slowly and gets worse over time. It takes away the person's ability to think, reason, remember and it interferes with a person's daily life and activities.

In this situation it is important that you understand that your loved one is helpless, and unable to control this behavior. Even though there will be moments when you feel

Alzheimer's Tips You Should Know

certain that they know what they are doing because they seem to wait until you turn your back or move away to spit, truth is they are not in control. They are not trying to make your life miserable, or to make you unhappy. That is the first thing you need to remember.

As you read along, you will learn why your loved one is spitting and we will offer strategies to cope with the issue.

WHY HAS YOUR LOVED ONE SUDDENLY STARTED SPITTING

We cannot explore the problems of spitting in Alzheimer's patients, without considering the effects that the disease has on the person's ability to swallow, and how this in turn creates what we may consider a spitting dilemma for the caregiver.

"FORGETTING" TO SWALLOW

As the disease progresses, memory loss occurs not only in the memory and thinking centers, but also in the physical parts of the body.

Alzheimer's Tips You Should Know

Normally, the function of swallowing just happens; it is something that we do without thought or effort. Generating and swallowing saliva for a person without the disease is automatic and we are not even aware when we are doing so. That's because our bodies are functioning as normal.

When we have food, drink or even saliva to swallow, the brain sends a message from its swallowing center, letting our body know that there is something to be swallowed, and in normal cases we do so automatically. However, the problem in the case of Alzheimer's disease is that the brain is damaged and as a result, that message may be faulty or may not even get through at all. The end result is that your loved one "forgets to swallow" as the message was ineffective.

So as this action is no longer automatic, you will find that rather than swallow the saliva, your loved one will either spit it out every time, anywhere, or they will accumulate all that saliva for some time and then expel it from their mouth when they feel to.

The retention of saliva should be monitored carefully as your loved one can either choke on it, or it may leak into their lungs, eventually causing pneumonia.

BOREDOM

Is your loved one bored or anxious? Consider whether these may be the reason why they are spitting. Everyone hates boredom, even a person with Alzheimer's disease. If your loved one is sitting around all day long with little or no activity to stimulate their senses, then it is quite likely that this may be the reason.

MEDICATION

The use of certain medications may be the reason why your loved one is spitting. Consult your doctor about this as a possible trigger.

JUST ANOTHER UNEXPLAINABLE BEHAVIOR

In many cases, spitting in a person with Alzheimer's disease may be just another dysfunctional behavior which occurs. Persons with Alzheimer's disease can present with several types of unusual behavior. Some may tear anything that they can, tie knots in curtains, flush objects down the toilet, eat anything that is edible including feces and engage in many other behaviors that are hard to explain. Some of these behaviors including spitting may last for a long time or may start and stop suddenly. Unfortunately these types of behaviors are not easy to stop or control and do not respond to pharmotherapeutic management.

HOW TO COPE WITH THE SPITTING PROBLEM

Alzheimer's Tips You Should Know

I wish that I could wave a magic wand and give you a simple solution, to a problem that I prayed would just go away. One day without warning, out of the blue, my mother who has been living with Alzheimer's disease for nine years started spitting suddenly. Honestly, it really irritated me and I tried and tried all types of stuff, like offering a towel to spit in instead of on the floor, placing a bucket or cup close by, and even placing a towel around the areas where she sat. All of this was fruitless, because she would fold up the towel, play with the bucket and eventually walk around and spit everywhere.

Dealing with this dilemma could be a battle with fire or it could be a time where you grow in virtues and character. It will take an enormous amount of love, patience and tolerance, but also a little creativity. Remember, that Alzheimer's disease affects each person differently so what works for one person may not work for another.

Alzheimer's Tips You Should Know

ACCEPTANCE

I spent many weeks in agony, throwing my hands in the air and fussing, searching everywhere hoping to find a simple answer, maybe a pill, a spitting deterrent or anything that would ease my pain, but to no avail.

Then suddenly like a bolt of lightning, I was struck with the realization that my biggest problem was not my mother and the spitting but it was actually me. Here I was, asking my mum who was dealing with a disease that had damaged her brain and changed her whole life, to stop spitting everywhere and I actually expected that she would listen. I smile as I write this part, because I was supposed to be the person who was well. My greatest release came when I accepted the fact, that my mother just could not help it and that I was the one who had to change my attitude towards the situation. As I accepted that, mopping, wiping and cleaning became much easier. It reduced my stress, caused me to be happier and reduced the tension when the spitting began.

BLAME IT ON AL

Even after accepting the fact that my mother was helpless. There were times when the toll of cleaning spit twenty times or more in one hour became too much. Times when I still felt irritated, upset and defeated. In those moments though, because of my acceptance, I now put the blame not to my mother but on Alzheimer's disease. As a result I was able to be more compassionate and tolerant about what was happening.

I cannot emphasize enough the fact, that if life is to be easier for you and your loved one you need to look inward.

No amount of shouting yelling, or cursing will stop them from spitting on the floor or walls. As a matter of fact, it will only create a threatening environment, which will in turn cause aggression and fear in your loved one. Then the situation becomes worse.

Alzheimer's Tips You Should Know

I encourage you most of all, therefore, to see your mother, father, sister, friend, husband or wife or whoever you are caring for, through eyes of compassion and love.

KEEP YOUR LOVED ONE ACTIVE

Talk

A build -up of saliva in the mouth of your loved one is almost impossible, if they are engaged in conversation.

Of course, they cannot talk, talk, talk all day long but having conversations, singing songs and finding time for stimulating activities can ease the spitting dilemma.

In the later stages of the disease, your loved one may lose the ability to communicate verbally and find difficulty expressing their thoughts and feelings Their words may become jumbled and this may make communicating with them difficult. However, this does not mean that communication should cease altogether.

Talk about things they loved to do in the past, people they enjoyed sharing with, hobbies, or current affairs, whatever makes them happy. Ask questions and give them opportunity to respond, even though you may not understand, their attempt to answer may release accumulated saliva in the mouth. However, if you find that your loved one is becoming agitated either change the conversation or try again later. Although I could not understand what my mother was saying, our discussions would often be about her mum, her grandfather and her grandmother. Why? These were the people whom she would respond positively to when you mentioned there name and at times she would even start a conversation and ask questions. Even though I could not understand, I responded saying things like "Yes, granddaddy loved to cook lots of food for you" and then follow up with a question like "Did you like your granddaddy's food a lot?" and she would respond in some way. That's why I encourage you to keep talking about positive things and people, recall stories that they would have told you and discuss them. Even though neither of you may understand, it will also be good for the relationship.

Go outdoors

Going out doors with your loved one sometimes is a good idea. Of course you should always be aware that they should not be left alone. Going outdoors is not only good for the change of environment and stimulating your loved ones senses but it also takes the spit out doors. If you are going for a walk, avoid crowded areas, or you may just want to sit outdoors in the patio or on a bench in the park where your loved one cannot spit on any one.

If you must go to a restaurant ask for a table that is away from others or instead of restaurants try having picnics.

Outdoor activities will reduce the amount of mopping that you would have to do and could very well reduce the desire to spit. Your loved one will be stimulated by the environment. The touch of leaves or other safe surfaces will also be good for them, at least it will get them out of the house and busy. Of course, you must take care that you do not let them out of your sight, as they may wander away.

Use their favorite foods and snacks

Stimulate their sense of taste. Monitor your loved one, when you notice that they are retaining saliva in their mouth; offer them something that they enjoy eating, not in large quantities, but enough to get them chewing every now and then. They will either swallow the saliva along with the food, spit it out where you can see, or it will drool out as they open their mouth to bite.

Try some hard candy or mints for them to suck on during the day. Be very careful not to use candy that can be a choking hazard. Use their favorite flavors and do not give them the wrappers, as they may mistakenly place them in their mouths as well.

Cue your loved one to swallow

The accumulation of saliva in the mouth can become dangerous for persons who have Alzheimer's disease, as it can cause choking or aspiration pneumonia. **Aspiration pneumonia** occurs when foreign matter such as food, vomit and even saliva leaks into your lungs allowing bacteria to enter and causing severe lung infection. Persons with Alzheimer's disease are susceptible to aspiration pneumonia, because the damage to the brain causes them to "forget to swallow" and also affects their swallowing reflexes.

In cases where your loved one is not aggressive and agitated you can "cue" or "remind" them to swallow, by gently moving the persons chin in a chewing motion to get it started, or by gently stroking the throat to encourage swallowing.

Verbally cue your loved one to spit

Since the accumulation of saliva in the mouth is potentially dangerous for your loved one, it is important that you do not ignore it. It may become necessary to verbally cue your loved one to spit out the saliva. Do not shout. Try taking them to the sink and repeat "SPIT! SPIT! SPIT!" You may need to repeat this several times before they respond positively.

It is a good idea to invest in a manual saliva suction pump. This is very useful in instances where you are unable to get your loved one to spit willingly. In this case you have to manually pump the saliva from the mouth.

When your loved one spits at you and others

As Alzheimer's disease progresses, mainly in the later stages of the illness, your loved one may exhibit aggressive behavior which may include biting, hitting, screaming and scratching. Spitting at others is also included in this type of *behavior.*

As a caregiver, family member or friend you need to understand that this type of behavior is not uncommon with Alzheimer's disease. So you may find that a person, who was quite mild-mannered and pleasant, may throw you some surprises, by exhibiting behaviors and actions that they would never have done before.

Remember, this disease damages the brain and eventually affects every area of the person's life and functions. Personality changes, loss of inhibition and self- control and emotional discomfort, may cause your loved one to become aggressive and even spit at caregivers, family friends and others.

Another point to consider is whether there is emotional or physical discomfort that may cause the aggression or unusual behavior such as spitting.

Do not take it personally

Spitting at you and aggression in any form, can be upsetting, but the most important thing to remember, is that the person is NOT doing it deliberately. Even though it may appear that the behavior is targeted at you, do not take it personally, it may be just that you are the person there at that time. The fact that the person is aggressive to you does not mean that their feelings have changed towards you or that they hate you. Remember, there is damage to the brain and other changes are taking place as a result. Chances are that the same loved one, who may have spat on or at you, this moment, will respond positively towards you a few minutes later. With Alzheimer's disease a person's mood can change in a twinkling of an eye.

As dementia slowly robs your loved one of self-awareness, the person becomes less inhibited, losing both the memory of how he or she once behaved, as well as a sense of social norms. As a result of this, your loved one may undress in public, say inappropriate things (rude comments, cursing), stare at strangers, and may also spit at others.

There are no simple answers to dealing with these types of behaviors and it can make caregiving even more difficult. However, through a gradual process of identifying what might have triggered the spitting or other unusual behavior, you may be able to deal with it appropriately.

What may cause your loved one to spit at others?

Remember that all behaviors are a way of communicating. They may be feeling frustrated, under pressure, or humiliated, because they no longer have the ability to cope with the everyday demands of life.

They may feel that there is an invasion of their privacy or that their independence is threatened. For example, a person who has to be assisted with bathing may resist and exhibit aggressive behavior by spitting at the caregiver. This may happen as said earlier, because the person feels that their privacy is being invaded, or they might even see you as a stranger.

Being in an unfamiliar environment, where there is too much noise, or too many people around, can make them confused and anxious. In this case your loved one may get nervous and feel threatened, especially if they do not recognize the people around them. As a result, they may react inappropriately by spitting at others in protest.

Alzheimer's Tips You Should Know

Even in the home environment, persons with Alzheimer's disease may mistake plants, pictures and even you for a stranger or a robber and become aggressive and exhibit behavior that you may find unusual, but to them, it is a way of protecting themselves.

Your loved one may be dealing with physical discomfort or pain; may be bored, or even simply thirsty. However, they are unable to communicate these emotions in a way that we consider to be socially acceptable.

Are you shouting, quarrelling or being aggressive towards your loved one. If so spitting at you may be a response to your own aggression.

How to respond to spitting and other unusual behaviors

If your loved one is behaving rudely by spitting, insulting people or swearing – do not start arguing and shouting in an attempt to correct the behavior. This will only agitate the situation. Try to distract your loved one's attention, apologize and explain to the people affected, that the behavior is due to Alzheimer's disease and is not directed at them personally.

If the behavior occurs in the home, take a deep breath, step away from the person, and clean yourself off. Though, it is upsetting, try to see it through the eyes of compassion, and remember that it is not something that will kill you.

Being spat on can easily upset you as the caregiver. You may feel that you want to respond in like manner. Try to stay calm, do not argue, and do not strike back. If you respond in like manner, the situation may escalate and you on reflection will be sorry that you did. If the behavior occurs in the home, take a deep breath, step away from the person and give them space. The person with Alzheimer's disease can change moods quickly, so the time away will allow you and them to calm down.

Ask yourself if what you are trying to do for the person must be done at that time. If it can be put off, do so and come back in a few minutes, you will be surprised what a difference it can make.

Being spat on can be humiliating, may hurt your feelings, and can leave you feeling upset and timid to go back and help your loved one for fear that it will happen again. However, you will need to find ways to help yourself recover after the incident. Your loved one needs your help, love and compassion.

Make every effort not to become resentful and recognize that the incident may occur again. As noted earlier, your outlook and attitude towards the situation will be the key in how you handle it. Get support from friends, family or members of your church or other faith groups.

You may have lost your temper, do not allow guilt to control you, look forward to handling the situation better the next time, if it does occur again.

Alzheimer's Tips You Should Know

Always deal with any personal issues that may be affecting you before you attend to your loved one. If you are already angry about some other situation, it is more likely that if your loved one spits on you, that you will respond angrily.

Love and compassion are the key attributes needed to take care of your loved one. At every stage the person with Alzheimer's disease will exhibit different behaviors and actions. Functions that they could perform before will be impossible for them to do now. Words that they could speak may become extinct. Their brain has been damaged by the disease and they can no longer control certain behaviors.

When your loved one is spitting out food and drink

There are times when the person may spit out food or drink either immediately or they may pocket some in their cheeks and spit it out later. This may be happening for a number of reasons.

SWALLOWING DISORDERS

All spitting issues are not because of "forgetting to swallow". Caregivers and families should observe their loved ones carefully, to see whether they are encountering problems swallowing.

Dysphagia

Dysphagia is the term used for difficulty swallowing. In the late stages of Alzheimer's disease, your loved one may experience this problem. As the disease continues to damage the brain, it also extends to the entire body, including the ability to swallow when the muscles and the swallowing reflexes deteriorate.

Perhaps, you have realized a hoarse voice, recurrent hiccupping, and the deep cough in your loved one. Maybe they are pocketing food in their cheeks and then spitting it out, or even spitting it out as soon as it is placed in the mouth. If these things are happening, it may be a sign of dysphagia.

As soon as you notice these signs it is important to consult the doctor. In some instances, the person may be at the end-of-life stage and the body's systems may be starting to shut down and eating and drinking may no longer be desired. Your doctor should be able to guide you through this stage.

It is important that you pay close attention to your loved one at mealtime. You should not just place the meal on the table for your loved one to manage. Even without swallowing difficulties, this approach is not advised, as there are other issues that Alzheimer's patients are faced with at mealtime, due to cognitive decline. In many instances, your loved one may not be able to

Alzheimer's Tips You Should Know

interpret that the meal is actually there to be eaten. As a result some people with Alzheimer's disease may become malnourished, or dehydrated, because they are no longer able to manage their mealtime and feed themselves.

Ensure that your loved one is comfortable when they are seated to eat. Use devices and cushions that would keep the person in an upright position. This is important so that they do not slide down in the chair. Gently position the head forward.

After eating, keep the person in an upright sitting position for about 30 minutes.

If your loved one has reached the stage where the swallowing of liquids is problematic, then you can add over-the-counter thickening powders to drinks, soups and other liquids.

In some instances, you can also add rice cereals or oatmeal to milk to increase its thickness. Make sure that you do not add too

Alzheimer's Tips You Should Know

much, because you do not want to make it so thick, that it becomes a solid. You can thicken juices also, by adding pureed fruit, again in small amounts to avoid too much thickness. Cut solid foods in very small pieces and add gravies and sauces to foods for lubrication, which will make it easier to swallow.

Give your loved one enough time to eat their meals. Always make sure that you have enough time to spend with your loved one at mealtime without having to rush. Also do not force or rush your loved one. Try to allow at least one hour for meals.

Your loved one may not be able to eat the same quantities of food all at once, like they did before. In this case, you may need to divide the meals in smaller portions.

"Forgetting" what to do with the food

Your loved one may be at a stage where they may "forget" what is to be done with the food or even saliva in their mouth and there may just spit out thinking that it does not belong there. This happens as the disease progresses because the systems in the brain that control automatic swallowing are damaged and ineffective.

If this is happening you should consult your doctor. You may also be able to remind" them to swallow, by gently moving the person's chin in a chewing motion to get it started and prompting them by saying in simple instructions "chew now" and "swallow now" , or by gently stroking the throat to encourage swallowing.

What I have found in my journey with Alzheimer's disease, is, that when we recognize and accept that our loved one has been afflicted by a disease, which causes them to do things they would never have normally, then cleaning moms pooh becomes an act of love rather than a dreaded task.

Alzheimer's Tips You Should Know

The difference between success and failure is attitude.

A Note from the Author

My journey with Alzheimer's disease began several years ago when my mother started asking the same question over and over again, making allegations about theft and behaving strangely. At that time I knew very little about the disease, or, that it would change our lives forever: but as they say "Experience is the greatest teacher"

It is a journey that is unchartered, filled with days of pain and challenges, but also days when you and your loved one can still create moments of joy. This book "Alzheimer's Tips You Should Know" is dedicated to all those

who have committed to providing care for
persons with Alzheimer's disease.

Safe Journey

A.V.Blackman

www.ingramcontent.com/pod-product-compliance
Lightning Source LLC
Chambersburg PA
CBHW060456290526
45791CB00001B/139